Pain-Free Sitting, Standing, and Walking

Pain-Free Sitting, Standing, and Walking

ALLEVIATE CHRONIC PAIN BY RELEARNING NATURAL MOVEMENT PATTERNS

Craig Williamson, MSOT

Shambhala

BOSTON & LONDON

2013

Shambhala Publications, Inc.
Horticultural Hall
300 Massachusetts Avenue
Boston, Massachusetts 02115
www.shambhala.com

The information in this book is not intended as a substitute for person-
alized medical advice. The reader should consult a physician before
beginning this or any exercise program. If you experience increased
pain during or after these exercises, it may indicate a problem that
requires the attention of your physician.

9 8 7 6 5 4 3 2 1

First Edition
Printed in the United States of America

♾ This edition is printed on acid-free paper that meets the American
National Standards Institute z39.48 Standard.
♻ This book is printed on 30% postconsumer recycled paper.
For more information please visit us at www.shambhala.com.
Distributed in the United States by Random House, Inc.,
and in Canada by Random House of Canada Ltd

Library of Congress Cataloging-in-Publication Data

Williamson, Craig.
Pain-free sitting, standing, and walking: alleviate chronic pain by
relearning natural movement patterns / Craig Williamson.
p. cm.
ISBN 978-1-59030-971-1 (pbk. : alk.paper)
1. Myalgia-Treatment. 2. Exercise therapy. I. Title.
RC935.M77W552012
616.7'42—dc23
2012025190

Dedicated to Adele and Paul Williamson

Contents

Acknowledgments

I HAD the good fortune to have artists help me complete this book. Thank you to photographers Troy Lucia and Nora Lindsay for your masterful skill and patience in producing the photographs. Thank you to artist Kirsten Moorhead for your expert anatomical drawings and clarity of vision. Thank you to mime-dancer Karen Montanaro for modeling the exercises, and for being Karen Montanaro. Thank you to poet Jonathan Weinert for your brilliant way with words.

To my clients and students who continue to teach me so much, thank you. To my supportive and encouraging friends near and far, I can't thank you enough. And as always, thank you to my family

Pain-Free Sitting, Standing, and Walking

Introduction

YOU PROBABLY already know how to sit, stand, and walk, but if you are uncomfortable when you do so, then you may need to take a closer look at how you perform these everyday movements. By practicing the exercises in this book, you can retrain your muscles to carry your body more efficiently and become aware of which muscle habits work and which do not. Muscle habits, sometimes called movement patterns, become dysfunctional when the muscles are habitually overworked or underworked. My book *Muscular Retraining for Pain-Free Living* explores movement patterns, carriage, and muscle pain in detail. It gives a good background for understanding the bigger picture of muscular retraining, but you do not need to read it to benefit from this book.

We are all so used to the familiar feeling of how we carry our bodies that we are often largely unaware of it. This is especially true of how we sit, stand, and walk, because we do these things automatically all day long. Many of us have developed dysfunctional movement patterns that do not allow us to sit, bend, crawl, squat, stand, walk, and run in the pain-free way we did as young children.

Your body is designed and programmed to move easily. Regardless of what has happened in your life, the memory of pain-free movement is still within you. You can tap into this memory by practicing natural movement patterns. The exercises described in this book will systematically retrain your muscles and improve your carriage.

The movement explorations and exercises let you feel ways of moving that are not your everyday muscle habits. When I am helping someone with sitting, standing, or walking, they often say something like, "Show me how to do it," or "Tell me what to do." My job is not to show you how to do it but to help you feel movement in a new way so that you learn to listen to your senses, which tell you when you are moving correctly. This kind of learning is not a process of imitation but of reconnecting with your body's feeling intelligence, the part of you that already knows how to move.

KINESTHETIC AWARENESS

Learning to carry your body with good alignment involves having normal kinesthetic awareness. *Kinesthesia* literally means "movement feeling." *Kinesthetic dysfunction* is the term I use to describe when someone does not accurately sense effort and relaxation in the muscles. Chapter 2 of *Muscular Retraining for Pain-Free Living* is devoted to this phenomenon. If you are not familiar with kinesthetic dysfunction, I encourage you to read it.

Muscular retraining *is* kinesthetic retraining. Muscles function based on the available kinesthetic awareness. As you practice the exercises in this book, remember that your kinesthetic awareness allows you to improve how you carry yourself, how you use your muscles, and your capacity to relax your muscles.

PAIN AND EMOTIONS

The body, mind, and psyche are not separate from each other. Because we have been heavily conditioned to think otherwise, we can become confused when it comes to interpreting physical pain. Pain is one way you get information, not just about your body, but also about your mind and psyche. In other words, pain helps you find out something about yourself.

Psychogenic pain—actual physical pain that has a psychological origin—is commonplace. The root of such pain is the unconscious capacity to repress thoughts and feelings, which prevents you from being aware of their existence. In the same way that you can be unaware of kinesthetic feelings, you can also be unaware of emotional feelings.

The subject of psychogenic pain is beyond the scope of this book, but it is tremendously important. The mind and psyche are rarely absent from chronic pain problems and are often at the bottom of them. Don't let your practice of corrective exercises fool you into thinking that the cause of your pain is purely physical. Few health issues are purely physical, because the body, mind, and psyche are interdependent. If you do not keep this fact in mind, the exercises you do may distract you from becoming aware of unconscious thoughts and feelings that are trying to get your attention through your pain. It is important to consider the role of repressed emotions and undermining thoughts in any ongoing pain problem.

How to Work with the Exercises in This Book

The exercises and explorations in this book are not arranged in order of difficulty but in the sequence that I have found best for learning. You may find some of the exercises very easy and others more challenging. The goal is to help you find a comfortable way to carry yourself when you sit, stand, and walk. As that happens, your reliance on the exercises will gradually lessen. If you experience pain in the future, particular exercises may help you remember important points you have forgotten. Or, like many people, you may no longer need to do the exercises at all, because what you have learned will be reinforced whenever you sit, stand, or walk.

To make this material easier to learn, I make a distinction between an *exploration* and an *exercise*. The explorations are intended to help you discover some of the building blocks of the various exercises. You should practice the exercises regularly until you find them easy. There is considerable overlap between explorations and exercises, because they all involve using kinesthetic awareness to reinforce new movement patterns. If you find any of the explorations to be as helpful as an exercise, then practice those regularly along with the other exercises. If an exploration is particularly relevant to an exercise, it is referred to as a *prerequisite* at the beginning of the exercise, but assume that each exercise and exploration is a prerequisite for the exercises that follow. Photographs of the basic positions for each exploration can be found in the appendix of this book.

The description of each exercise includes a recommended number of repetitions of the movement. If doing more than that number helps you learn the movement, then do more. Keep in mind, it is your awareness that facilitates learning new muscle habits, so mindful repetition is important.

I have found that inalterable teaching methods can limit the learning process. My goal as a teacher is for you to learn helpful information and to learn *how* to learn. Everyone has a unique way of learning and understanding. Whenever I work with clients and students, I continuously encourage them to make discoveries for themselves. Some of my favorite exercises are those that were discovered when I watched clients "misinterpret" my exercise instructions. Thanks to their nonknowing, they stumbled on something new and better. Use the instructions in this book as guidelines but not as absolute rules.

A Word Regarding Painful Exercise
These explorations and exercises are meant to be painless. If you experience pain or discomfort with any of these movements, move more slowly and with less effort. Take the time to discover how to make the movement painless by relaxing any unnecessary tension within your body. If you still feel pain, then skip over that particular exercise.

Let's get started learning more comfortable ways of sitting, standing, and walking.

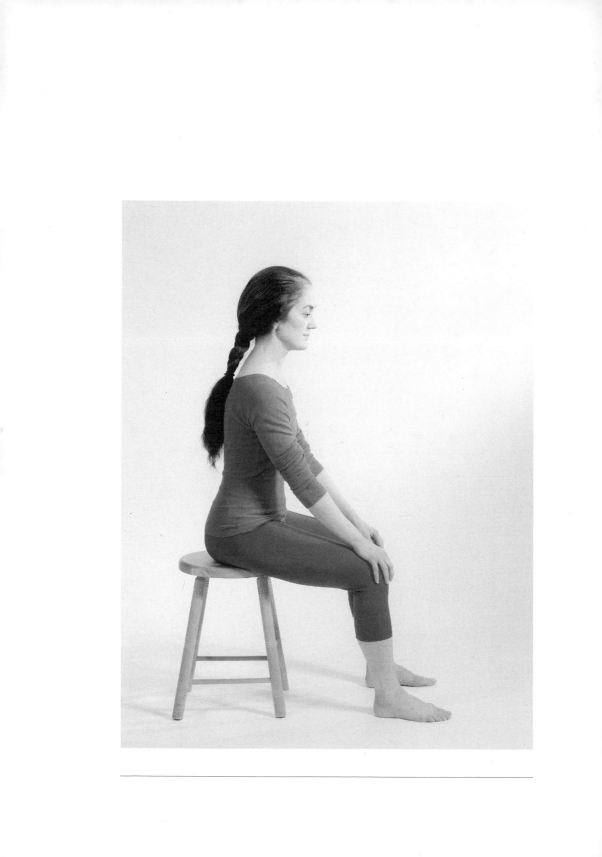

1 Sitting

SITTING is the most common activity in our society. Many of us spend most of the day in a seated position. It all begins when we ride around in car seats as babies and small children, followed by years of sitting in classrooms. As adults, many of us sit in cars or trains to get to work, sit all day on the job, and then sit on the way home again. At home, we sit in our easy chairs to relax from the day. One of the problems with all this sitting, as well as the predominantly mental activities in which we engage much of the time, is that body sense becomes dulled. I have worked with many clients who are largely unaware of their body, until pain reminds them of it. This may have become the norm for our culture, but it is not natural.

We need to take a look at *how* we sit, which includes how we perceive ourselves as we sit. Many people do not perceive sitting as an activity. For example, when you walk, your body is active, and when you sleep, your body is inactive. What about sitting? Is it an activity or more like sleeping?

If you consider sitting an activity, then you will be more aware of how you carry yourself. I prefer to use the word *carriage* instead of *posture*, because carrying yourself is an action that occurs moment to moment. It is something that involves your conscious participation.

Why go to the trouble of becoming aware of how you carry yourself? Two compelling reasons are to be more comfortable and to breathe better. There is also a broader, existential reason: since your body, mind, and psyche are interconnected, your carriage affects how you feel and is affected by your feelings. Being aware of how you carry yourself is another way to know yourself, because this awareness is part of your sense of who you are from moment to moment. An unmistakable sense of well-being comes from carrying yourself comfortably. It does not solve all your problems; in fact, it may not specifically solve any of them. Yet it helps you be present in your mind and psyche, which is of fundamental importance to your well-being.

To relearn your innate sense of carriage, you need to be aware of what is happening in your body. In practical terms, this means understanding the basic anatomy involved and being able to feel how your muscles and bones move, work, and relax. This is not magic; it is common sense. Actually, there is a little magic involved—the magic of your kinesthetic awareness that shows you how to carry yourself the easy way.

A Brief Overview of the Pelvis and Spine

The pelvis has left and right halves that are joined to the lowest part of the spine, which is called the *sacrum*. Each half of the pelvis is made up of three different bones that become fused in adulthood: the *ilium*, the *ischium*, and the *pubic bone* (figure 1.1).

When you sit in a chair, the part of your pelvis that is in contact with the seat comprises the *ischial tuberosities*, which are commonly referred to as the sit bones. In figure 1.1, you can see that the sit bones have a rounded shape, similar to the rockers on a rocking chair. Notice the prominence on each sit bone and that, in front of the prominence, the bones are fairly flat (the *inferior ischial ramus*). This flat area is the part of the sit bone that needs to be on the seat if you want your pelvis and lumbar spine to be in good alignment.

The sacrum can be considered part of the pelvis or part of the spine. When you sit in a chair, your pelvis is your base, and your spine extends upward out of this base. This means that the angle of the pelvis always

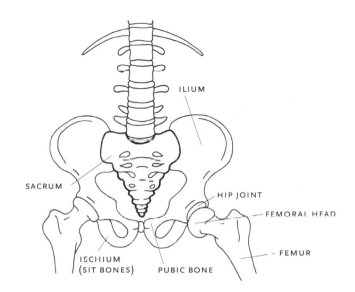

SACRUM

ILIUM

HIP JOINT

FEMORAL HEAD

FEMUR

ISCHIUM
(SIT BONES)

PUBIC BONE

Fig. 1.1

affects the alignment of the spine. Therefore, the most fundamental thing you can do for the alignment of your spine is to position your pelvis correctly.

The pelvis and spine are part of the area referred to as the trunk of the body. Technically, the trunk is the combination of the pelvis, abdomen, back, and chest.

When the pelvis is carried properly, the lumbar spine is able to maintain its natural curve, whether you are sitting, standing, or walking. When viewed from behind, the lumbar curve is concave (arcs inward). The entire structure of the lumbar spine includes discs, joints, ligaments, and bones, which function best when the lumbar curve is present. Prolonged flattening of this curve will distort the structures of the spine, which can lead to pain. To keep or regain your natural lumbar curve, you need to carry your pelvis correctly.

The easiest way to begin learning how to carry your pelvis and lumbar spine is by feeling how they function while you are sitting in a chair. What you learn from sitting also holds true for standing and walking.

The following explorations will give you a reliable way to sense and find the natural tilt of your pelvis.

≟ Sitting Exploration 1

- Sit on a chair with a firm seat whose height places your pelvis at least as high as your knees.

- Before getting started, let's clarify what we mean by tilting the pelvis either forward or backward. If I ask you to tilt your pelvis forward, I mean that you should tilt *the top of your pelvis*, just below your waist, forward. If I ask you to tilt your pelvis backward, I mean that you should tilt *the top of your pelvis* backward. About half the people I teach initially think that tilting forward is really tilting backward and vice versa. I use this terminology repeatedly throughout the book, so make sure you know its correct meaning.

- First, tilt of your pelvis backward. Think of it as a ball that is rolling toward the back of the seat.

- Next, tilt your pelvis forward, as if it were a ball rolling toward the front of the seat. Continue to tilt slowly backward and forward and observe what happens in other parts of your body as you do so.

- When you tilt your pelvis backward, notice how your head drops down and your chest caves in. The curve of your lower back is reversed because the weight on your pelvis is now behind your sit bones. Feel how your back muscles relax when your head and chest are slumped forward.

- When you tilt your pelvis forward, notice how your chest and head come up automatically, without you pulling your shoulders back. The chest and head come up as the lumbar curve increases.

≟ Sitting Exploration 2

- Begin by reviewing figure 1.1 to see where the sit bones are on the pelvis, and notice where the prominence of each sit bone is.

As already mentioned, the section of the sit bone in front of the prominence is fairly straight and flat. In this exploration, you will sense how it feels to sit on different parts of your sit bones and how that affects the posture of your back.

- Tilt your pelvis backward and forward, as in Exploration 1. As you do this, sense the weight and pressure of your sit bones against the chair seat. There will be one place where your weight feels most concentrated on each sit bone. That is the point at which you are directly over the bony prominence of each sit bone.

- As you tilt your pelvis backward, feel how your weight goes behind the bony prominence. If you exaggerate this movement, you will eventually be sitting on your tailbone.

- As you tilt your pelvis forward, feel how your weight will again pass over the bony prominence. If you continue to tilt beyond the prominence, you will be sitting on the flat section in the front of each sit bone.

⸗ Sitting Exploration 3

- Now let's find a comfortable sitting position. First, sit with your weight on the bony prominences of your sit bones. Tilt your pelvis forward a little bit until you can feel your weight on the flat bones in front of the prominence, which will feel like small platforms. It is easy to sit on the front of your sit bones because the area is flat.

- Notice the curve in your lower back as you sit on the front of your sit bones; your lumbar spine is automatically in its natural curve. Think of this as your home base for sitting. It is an easy way to reestablish the feeling of your natural lumbar curve.

- Continue to sit on the front of your sit bones for another minute or two. Be aware of the positioning of your chest and head. Is it any different than usual? Imagine you are carrying the sky on top of your head. Experiment with how much you can relax your back and abdominal muscles while remaining on the front of your sit bones. The more aligned your pelvis and spine are, the less work your back and abdominal muscles need to do.

- I call this pelvic position the "neutral tilt position," meaning the amount of tilt in the pelvis that provides the most support for the spinal curves and the carriage of the head. Some people have been taught (incorrectly) that the neutral tilt of the pelvis is found by sitting on the bony prominences of the sit bones, but that is actually a backward tilt.

The Hip Joint

In the explorations you just tried, your pelvis tilted forward and backward while your legs remained stationary. You can do this because your hip joints are rounded. Each joint consists of a rounded indentation on the side of the pelvis; the ball-shaped top of the thighbone fits into this indentation (see figure 1.1). The thighbone is called the *femur*, and the ball-shaped top is called the *femoral head*. The important point to remember here is that the hip joint is rounded.

When you lift your leg, the femoral head rolls within the hip socket. Conversely, when you tilt your pelvis forward and backward, the hip sockets roll around the femoral heads. Because the hip joint is rounded, either the ball or the socket can roll in any direction. In sitting, the pelvis primarily tilts forward and backward from the hips. In walking, the pelvis moves in all directions, as we will explore further in Chapter 3.

When you tilt your pelvis forward and backward, your hip joints move like hinges. Each hinge folds closed when the pelvis tilts forward and opens when it tilts backward (see figures 1.2–1.5). Many adults have forgotten the feeling of how their hip joints are supposed to move. This loss of kinesthesia is a serious concern, because the hip joint is central to sitting, bending, standing, turning, and walking. Many of the explorations and exercises in this book will help you restore your kinesthetic awareness of your hip joints' hinge movement, as well as movement in other directions.

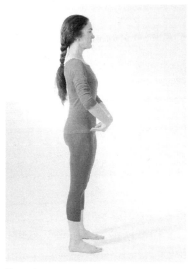

Fig. 1.2

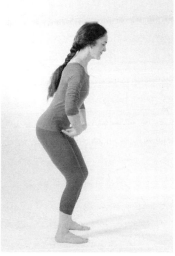

Fig. 1.3

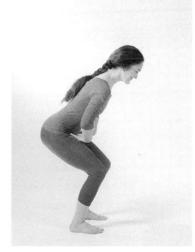

Fig. 1.4

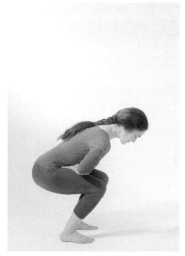

Fig. 1.5

The Iliacus and Psoas Muscles

The most important aspect of sitting is the position of your pelvis. Memorize this and then continue.

When you are sitting in a chair, gravity will cause your pelvis to tilt backward, not forward. But, as you discovered in the earlier explorations, you need to sit on the front part of your sit bones to have good spinal alignment. This means that you need to find a good way to prevent your pelvis from tilting backward when you are sitting.

It might seem like the solution is a well-designed chair, which can certainly be helpful, but no chair is going to do all the work for you. Leaning against the back of your chair will prevent your pelvis from tilting backward completely, but depending on the chair's design, it may still allow your pelvis to tilt enough to flatten your lumbar curve. Using a chair with a higher seat, so that your hips are higher than your knees, will encourage your pelvis to tilt forward, but it is still possible to slouch and tilt your pelvis backward. The ideal solution is to know how to use your body so you are not at the mercy of your chair. The starting point for this is sensing the action of the *iliacus* and *psoas* muscles.

Look at the drawing of the iliacus and psoas muscles in figure 1.6. The iliacus muscle connects the top of the inside of the femur (the lesser

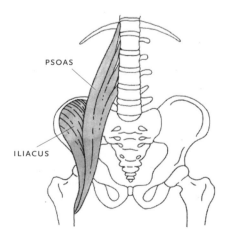

Fig. 1.6

trochanter) to the front of the pelvis (the ilium); the psoas muscle connects the top of the inside of femur (the lesser trochanter) to the sides (the transverse processes) of the five lumbar vertebrae. These two muscles are sometimes considered to be one (the *iliopsoas*), because they work together to raise the leg, a movement referred to as hip flexion. However, the term *iliopsoas* oversimplifies the functions of the iliacus and psoas muscles.

In *Muscular Retraining for Pain-Free Living*, I oversimplified this further by referring to the psoas and iliacus muscles together as the *psoas* in order to give a general idea of these muscles, but it is better to think of the iliacus and psoas muscles individually, because they have distinct functions. The iliacus muscle is fundamental to sitting, because it is perfectly placed to tilt the pelvis forward and, therefore, to prevent it from tilting backward. The psoas muscle is responsible for many things, including the natural lumbar curve. For the psoas to maintain the curve, the iliacus needs to be keeping the pelvis in the proper position.

If you are sitting on a stool without your iliacus and psoas muscles engaged, you will either (1) let your pelvis tilt backward, which causes your spine to slouch, or (2) try to prevent your pelvis from tilting backward by tensing your back muscles too much. Let's take a quick look at these two conditions.

Allowing your pelvis to tilt backward and your chest to slouch means relaxing your iliacus, psoas, and back muscles. This is what tends to happen if you are sitting back on a big overstuffed couch. Because your back muscles are relaxed in this position, it may feel comfortable. The problem comes from habitually sitting this way for years; it eventually compresses the structures of the lumbar spine. Another problem with this position is that it can interfere with breathing. Try it to find out.

Preventing your pelvis from tilting backward without the help of the iliacus and psoas muscles requires your back muscles to do all the work, which can become tiring. When these muscles are tired, a chair with lumbar support will give them some relief.

However, the best solution for sitting upright is to use your iliacus muscles to keep your pelvis tilted forward so that you are resting on the front of your sit bones and to use your psoas muscles to keep your natural lumbar curve. Your back muscles remain relatively relaxed yet still carry your spine in its natural shape.

⸗ Sitting Exploration 4

- Sit on the front half of a chair or stool. Place your feet flat on the ground, well in front of your knees. Tilt your pelvis backward so that your chest caves in and your head drops down. Relax your back muscles completely. Cross your arms over your chest or let them relax in your lap.

- The goal of this exploration is for you to be able to identify and engage the iliacus muscles, which are in the front of your pelvis, to tilt it forward. Throughout this exploration, your back will remain curved over in a fully relaxed position so that you won't use your back muscles to help tilt your pelvis forward.

- Slowly attempt to pick up both of your knees without lifting any part of your feet off the ground. You will quickly discover that you can't actually raise your knees if your feet stay on the ground, but the idea is to use the same muscles as you would *if* you were trying to raise your knees. If you imagine a heavy weight on your knees, it may help you get a better feeling for this. You will try to *almost* raise your knees. When you do this, can you feel your pelvis tilting forward? Can you sense the muscles in the front of your hips working? The iliacus muscles are among those you are feeling.

- If your pelvis is not tilting forward at all, then press your hands down on your knees while you push your knees up into your hands. The resistance will encourage your hip flexors to work harder to pull your pelvis forward. Alternatively, you can ask someone else to press down on your knees while you try it.

- Press your feet into the floor to tilt your pelvis backward and return to the starting position.

- Repeat the motion of slowly tilting your pelvis forward and backward many times. This should show you that you can tilt your pelvis forward by using muscles other than those in your back. Keep your back rounded and your head down, as if your pelvis and spine are one piece, to ensure that your back muscles stay relaxed. Continue attempting to localize your iliacus muscles as you practice the movement. As long as you can sense your pelvis being tilted forward by something in the lower front of your pelvis, you are on the right track. After practicing the exercises in this chapter, this action will become more obvious to you.

CARRIAGE OF THE HEAD

The muscle tone and movement of your body is greatly influenced by how you carry your head. Carrying your head comfortably will make it easier for your whole body to relax. The less work your neck muscles do to keep your head upright, the less work your other muscles have to do to keep the rest of your body upright.

During the previous three explorations, you could feel how the position of your pelvis affects the position of your head. Although you can feel this in any upright position, it is particularly easy when you are seated. When the pelvis tilts backward, the entire spine tends to cave in, which brings the head forward. If you sensed this in the previous explorations, you've got a head start in understanding one cause of neck and upper back pain in people who sit all day at work.

It is easy to see when someone is carrying his head too far forward (figure 1.8), which is far more common than being carried too far backward (figure 1.9). This will be covered in more detail in Chapter 2, which introduces the idea of a vertical axis in the body. Ideally, the head will be directly above the chest, not far out in front of it nor pulled back

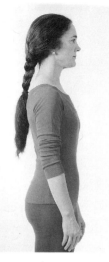

FIG. 1.7

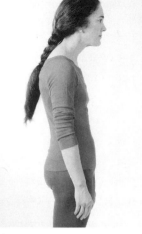

FIG. 1.8

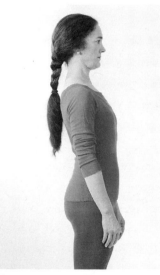

FIG. 1.9

too far (figure 1.7). When the head is carried too far in front of the chest, the neck slants forward. This forces the upper back and neck muscles to work harder to support the weight of the head, which in an adult is between eight and twelve pounds. However, if the head is carried directly above the chest, the neck is more vertical and therefore offers more support. The result is that the upper back and neck muscles work less.

Many people do exercises that pull their head backward to strengthen their neck muscles; they think that if their neck muscles are stronger, their head won't go forward. Some people follow this theory with such determination that they create upper back and neck tension by attempting to pull their head (and often their shoulders) backward all day long. I often suggest learning to relax the neck muscles, but I do not recommend trying to strengthen them. Toddlers do not have particularly strong necks, yet they able to carry their relatively big heads without a problem.

There is a difference between *strengthening* the neck muscles that pull your head backward and *sensing* that your head needs to be carried farther back. Mindfully moving your head backward while simultaneously tilting your pelvis forward can be useful, as you will see in Exercises 6 and 7 later in this chapter. This does not strengthen your neck, but it restores your kinesthetic sense of balancing your head on your neck. This feeling will teach you an easier way to carry your head.

The solution to a too-forward head posture begins with carrying the pelvis properly. This is not surprising if you look at the body as a whole, because the neck is the top of the spine, and the position of the spine depends on the position of the pelvis. When the pelvis is where it belongs, it is possible to improve the carriage of the head. For most people, this means that the head and neck will need to be carried farther backward than usual.

Your kinesthetic perception of your neck is greatly influenced by how you have been carrying it. If your neck muscles are tensed and compressed in the back, the front, or both, you will have the sense that your neck is shorter than it really is. This is because your head and upper neck have been moving as if they were one piece. On the other hand, if your neck muscles are relaxed and you carry your head naturally, you will perceive that your head is separate from your neck—which, of course, it is. Only then will you be able to sense the actual length of your neck.

The front of the neck is as long as the back. Who knew? Close your eyes for a moment and imagine the front of your neck going up as high as the back of your neck. The top of the neck is where the head rocks and pivots, roughly at the level of the nose and just below the ears, as shown in figure 1.10.

The benefit to being able to sense where your head moves on top of your spine is that your neck feels more relaxed and your head feels more upright. Remembering how long your neck really is helps improve

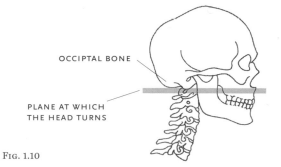

OCCIPITAL BONE

PLANE AT WHICH
THE HEAD TURNS

Fig. 1.10

how you carry your pelvis. How? It encourages your spine to maintain its natural curves, which in turn encourages your pelvis to remain in a neutral tilt. Good carriage of the head helps keep the pelvis better aligned and vice versa. You can observe this by feeling what happens in your neck when you look down. Do you tilt your pelvis backward every time you look down? This can be corrected by a better kinesthetic sense of how and where your skull moves on top of your neck. Exploration 5 will give you an opportunity to identify these sensations.

Look at figure 1.10 again, and notice the bone at the bottom of the back of the head. This is called the *occipital bone*. It is not only the back of the head, but also the underside of the back of the head, just behind the spine. When you touch the back of your head, you are touching the part of the occipital bone that faces directly behind you. You can't touch the underside of the occipital bone (which is just behind the spine), because it is covered by the many muscles that connect your neck to your head. When these muscles contract, the underside of the occipital bone (to which they attach) is pulled downward. As a result, the back of the neck is shortened.

Let's now explore how the neck carries the head.

⩰ Sitting Exploration 5

- Sit on the flat part of the front of your sit bones, as you did in the previous explorations. Look straight ahead. Hold this book in your lap, close to your pelvis.

- Look down at the book by leaning your whole neck far forward. Can you feel your pelvis tilt backward as your neck leans forward? Even if it is only a slight tilt backward, pay attention to this feeling as you keep looking up and down slowly a few more times.

- Look again at figure 1.10 to see where your head rests on top of your neck. Then imagine a line running from one earlobe to the other and passing through the joint between the top of your neck and the base of your head. Use this line to approximate where your head nods and turns at the top of your spine. Nod your head in tiny movements, slowly up and down, imagining and feeling the movement happening high on top of your neck.

- Now slowly look down at the book again. This time do not lean your neck forward. Imagine you are rolling your head over the top of your neck, as if you are rolling it over the edge of a high cliff. As you do this, intentionally remain seated on the front of your sit bones, and don't let your pelvis tilt backward. Look up again and repeat this many times, until you can clearly sense that your head can look downward without your pelvis tilting backward.

- Look straight ahead. Imagine a horizontal plane at the junction of your neck and your skull. Imagine this plane extending endlessly in every direction and your skull resting on it. Very slowly rotate your head to the left and then to the right. It does not matter how far you turn your head. Imagine that your head is turning itself without your neck making any effort, as if your neck is being pulled by your head. You can do this with your eyes open or closed. If your eyes are open, be aware of your wide peripheral vision as your head turns. Continue rotating your head slowly for 1 to 2 minutes.

- Look straight ahead. Imagine where the underside of your occipital bone is. This is the part of the bone that faces down, just behind your spine. Imagine that this entire flat surface is slowly floating upward. Just imagine it; don't make any muscular effort. Can you sense your lower back muscles adjusting as you do this? Finish this exploration by standing up and imagining the same thing. You may be able to sense your heels sinking deeper into the floor as you imagine the occipital bone floating upward.

The Back Muscles

The biggest complaint I hear from people about trying to sit upright all day at work is that it makes their back tired. So they end up slouching in their chair most of the time.

Many people conclude that their back is weak because it gets so tired when they try to sit upright. However, very few people have genuinely weak back muscles. There is nothing wrong with having strong back muscles, but superstrong back muscles are not necessary for pain-free sitting. More important than strong back muscles is a lack of unnecessary tension in those muscles. If you can sense movement at your hip joints, use your iliacus and psoas muscles to support your pelvis and lower spine, and balance your head on top of your neck, then you can minimize the work your back muscles need to do. As a result, your back muscles will be more relaxed in all of your activities.

Exercises that emphasize the use of your back muscles, such as Explorations 5 and 14 and Exercise 18, may feel good and leave you feeling more upright. Why? Because repeatedly engaging and relaxing your back muscles increases your kinesthetic sense of those muscles. As a result, you automatically use those muscles more efficiently, which makes it feel easier to stand upright. Because it feels easier, you may feel stronger. Technically, though, this would be an improvement in *muscle tone*, not an increase in strength. Muscle tone involves kinesthetic awareness and describes how tense or slack a muscle is; good muscle tone is halfway between tense and slack. Muscle tone is not the same as muscle strength. (To learn more about the difference between tone and strength, read *Muscular Retraining for Pain-Free Living*, pages 58–61.)

Movements that involve actively bending the spine forward, known as

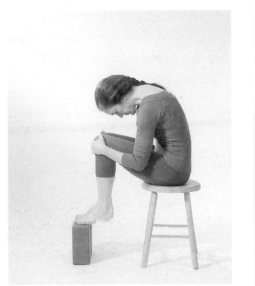

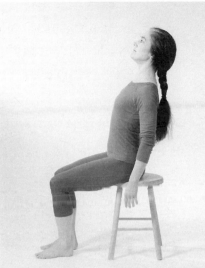

FIG. 1.11   FIG. 1.12

flexion, increase the tone of the abdominal muscles (figure 1.11). Movements that involve actively bending the spine backward, known as *extension,* increase the tone of the muscles that run vertically along each side of the spine (figure 1.12).

I have designed the exercises in this book to improve the tone of the muscles you need for sitting, standing, and walking. Many of these exercises involve back extension and flexion. If you are kinesthetically aware as you do a back extension exercise, the repeated action of bending backward and using your back muscles will help you feel more upright when you are sitting. There is no need, however, to continue the effort in those muscles after the exercise is over. If anything, hold on to the *feeling* of length in your spine that the exercise inspired.

⟳ Sitting Exploration 6

- Lie with your chest on the ground. Turn your head to the left or right, or else place one hand on top of the other and rest your forehead on top of your hands.

- Keeping your right leg straight, slowly raise it so that your knee is about five inches off the ground. Can you feel your lower back muscles working to lift your leg? You may also feel your middle and upper back muscles working. These are the back extensor muscles.

- Return your leg to the ground. Feel your back muscles relax. If they do not relax right away, then lie still until they do.

- Raise and lower your left leg in the same way. Imagine that you are initiating this movement from your back muscles rather than your leg muscles, as if your back is leading and your leg is following. Repeat lifting each leg until you can clearly sense your back muscles working and releasing.

KEY POINTS FOR SITTING

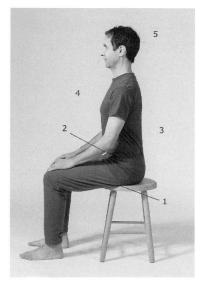

FIG. 1.13

1. Body weight rests on the front of the sit bones: Explorations 1–3; Exercise 5

2. The hip flexors are active: Exploration 4; Exercises 3–5

3. The back muscles are relaxed: Explorations 4 and 6; Exercises 1–5 and 8

4. The chest is open, and the shoulders are relaxed: Explorations 1–3; Exercises 5–8

5. The head is positioned directly over the upper body: Exploration 5; Exercises 6–8

Sitting Exercises

The first four sitting exercises begin on the floor, which is the best way to learn how to engage and release your lower back, abdominal, and hip flexor muscles. This will make the remaining exercises much easier.

1. Supine Lumbar Extension and Flexion

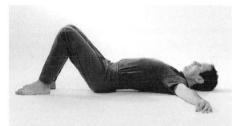

Fig. 1.14

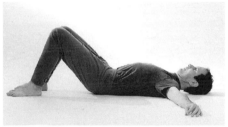

Fig. 1.15

Objective

To sense the relationship between the lower back and the abdominal muscles. When the lower back engages, the abdomen releases, and vice versa.

Position

▸ Lie on your back with your knees bent, your feet flat on the floor, and your legs and feet parallel to each other.

▸ Inhale and use your lower back muscles to exaggerate your lumbar curve, keeping your tailbone on the ground (figure 1.14). Relax your abdominal muscles. Inhale into your abdomen, using the breath to help you release your abdominal muscles.

▸ Next, exhale and use your abdominal muscles to press your lower back into the floor (figure 1.15). The curve of your lower back will flatten, and your tailbone will lift slightly off the floor.

▸ Continue moving back and forth slowly. Repeat the entire movement 8 times.

Sensing

Feel how your abdominal and lower back muscles work as partners in this movement. Notice that when your abdominals engage, your back muscles release, and vice versa. Imagine that your pelvis is like a ball, rolling down toward your feet and then up toward your head.

2. PELVIS LIFT WITH LEGS

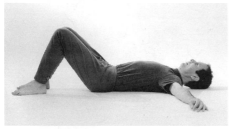 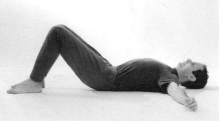

FIG. 1.16   FIG. 1.17

Prerequisite
Exploration 6

Objective
To be able to release the lower back muscles while using the legs, which retrains the lower back to relax.

Position
- Lie on your back with your knees bent, your feet flat on the floor, and your legs and feet parallel to each other (figure 1.16).
- Slowly press both of your feet into the floor, as if you were going to make an imprint of each foot in the floor. Allow your thighs to slide slightly toward your knees, as if each thigh were being pulled away from its hip socket. This small movement will lift your pelvis so that your tailbone is about two inches off the floor (figure 1.17). Relax your abdominal muscles *completely*—do not use them to tilt

your pelvis. Keep your lower back relaxed, so it drops into the floor, even as your pelvis tilts upward. The muscular effort for this motion comes only from your legs. If your lower spine lifts off the floor, you are either (1) not releasing your back muscles or (2) lifting your pelvis too high.

▸ Repeat this motion slowly 8 times.

▸ Some people find this exercise very easy, and there is no need to practice it further. However, if it seems difficult or impossible (which it may), practice this exercise every day until the coordination of these small, subtle movements becomes automatic.

Sensing

Feel how your lower back remains on the floor because you have allowed it to relax, not because you have pushed it down with your abdominal muscles.

3. Supine Hip Flexion

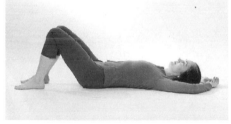
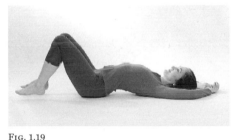

Fig. 1.18   Fig. 1.19

Prerequisite

Exploration 4

Objective

To be able to use the hip flexors without engaging the abdominal or lower back muscles. This exercise is directly applicable to sitting.

Position

▸ Lie on your back with your knees bent, your feet flat on the floor, and your legs and feet parallel to each other (figure 1.18).

▸ As you inhale, very slowly raise both of your feet a few inches off the ground. Relax your abdominal muscles and lower back muscles. This will cause the top front of your pelvis to roll toward your knees and your lumbar curve to increase (figure 1.19).

▸ As you exhale, return your legs to the starting position.

▸ Repeat 8 times.

Sensing

Feel the muscles at the top of the fronts of your legs cause your pelvis to roll forward. This exercise engages the iliacus and other muscles.

4. COMBINED HIP FLEXION AND PELVIS LIFT

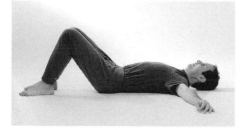

FIG. 1.20

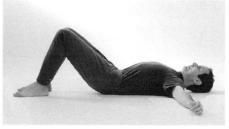

FIG. 1.21

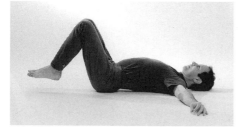

FIG. 1.22

Prerequisite
Explorations 4 and 6

Objective
To roll the pelvis back and forth without engaging the abdominal or lower back muscles. This retrains the lower back muscles to relax. This exercise is simply a combination of the previous two exercises.

Position
- Lie on your back with your knees bent, your feet flat on the floor, and your legs and feet parallel to each other (figure 1.20).
- Next, slowly press both of your feet into the floor, as if you were going to make an imprint of each foot in the floor. Allow your thighs to slide slightly toward your knees, as if each thigh were being pulled away from its hip socket. Your tailbone will lift about two inches off the floor, your lower back will drop down into the floor, and the front of your pelvis will move toward your head (figure 1.21). Relax your abdominal and lower back muscles completely. This is the same as Exercise 2.
- Return to the starting position (figure 1.20).
- Slowly raise both of your feet off the floor (figure 1.22). Relax your abdominal and lower back muscles. This will cause the front of your pelvis to move toward your knees and your lumbar curve to increase. This is the same as Exercise 3.
- Return to the starting position.
- Alternate between these two movements, keeping your abdominal and lower back muscles relaxed the entire time.
- Repeat 8 times.

Sensing
Feel how your pelvis rolls easily forward and backward, entirely from the use of your legs.

5. Seated Hip Flexion

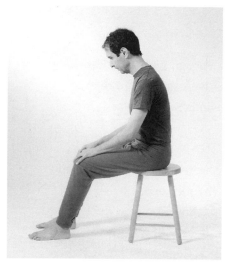

Fig. 1.23   Fig. 1.24

Prerequisites
Explorations 1–4

Objective
To fully use the iliacus muscles to sit with the weight on the front of the sit bones, maintaining the proper pelvic tilt.

Position
- Sit on the front half of a chair or stool. Place your feet flat on the floor, well in front of your knees (figure 1.23).
- Slowly attempt to *almost* lift your knees without lifting any part of your feet off the floor. Your knees can't go up if your feet stay down, but the goal is to have the top of your pelvis tilt forward from the effort of almost raising your knees. This activates the iliacus muscles.
- Tilt your pelvis forward until you are on the front of your sit bones. Your chest and head will become upright as your pelvis rolls forward (figure 1.24).
- Relax your hip muscles and return to the starting position.

- Keep your back muscles as relaxed as possible throughout this exercise; do not use them to tilt your pelvis forward. If your back muscles tense too much, it will interfere with the action of the iliacus muscles. If you have difficulty relaxing your back, try these techniques:
  - When you tilt the your pelvis forward, inhale into your abdomen (as in Exercise 1). This will help you relax your abdominal muscles. If you tense these muscles, it will prevent your pelvis from tilting forward.
  - When you tilt your pelvis forward, relax your shoulders.
  - When you tilt your pelvis forward, imagine your pubic bone moving toward the ground.
- Repeat 20 times.

Sensing

Feel how your pelvis tilts forward when you use the iliacus muscles. This is the main point of the exercise. The movement is an exaggeration of the iliacus action needed to sit on the front of your sit bones. Identify how much you can relax your back muscles yet still remain upright. You are sitting with your pelvis and lumbar spine in good alignment, supported by your hip flexors. This is the key to comfortable sitting.

6. PRONE NECK EXTENSION

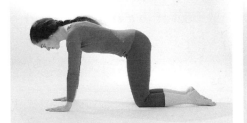

FIG. 1.25

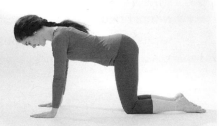

FIG. 1.26

Prerequisite
Exploration 5

Objective

To correct forward head posture.

Position

- ▸ Get on your hands and knees, with your face parallel to the ground and your hands directly below your shoulders.

Part One

- ▸ Relax your lower back, abdominal, chest, and shoulder muscles (figure 1.25). Gravity will encourage you to sense your lumbar curve without any lower back tension. Remain in this position for 30 seconds, or until your lower back feels relaxed.

Part Two

- ▸ Slowly raise the back of your head upward while keeping your face parallel to the ground; do not look up (figure 1.26). Keep your neck long; do not bunch up the muscles at the back of your neck. As you do this, *do not tighten the front of your shoulder or chest muscles*. In other words, your chest remains wide as you move your head up and down.
- ▸ Slowly return your head to the starting position.
- ▸ Repeat 8 times.

Sensing

Feel how your head can move backward while the back of your neck remains the same length. Also, sense how your head can be independent of your chest and shoulders, as evidenced by your ability to lift your head without tightening your chest or the front of your shoulders. In other words, you are not doing a push-up here.

7. Seated Neck Extension

Prerequisite

Explorations 1–5

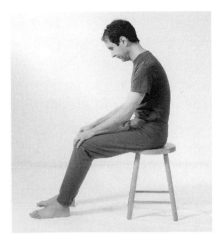 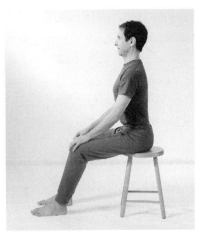

Fig. 1.27   Fig. 1.28

Objective

To sense the relationship between the forward pelvic tilt and the alignment of the head.

Position

- ▶ Sit with your upper body leaning a little forward, your chest caved in, and your head dropped forward. Relax your back muscles completely. Your hands can relax in your lap or on your knees (figure 1.27).
- ▶ Tilt your pelvis forward, as you did in Exercise 5. At the same time, shift your neck and head back and up, similar to the neck movement in Exercise 6. You will end up sitting on the front of your sit bones, with your head pulled back farther than normal. Your face should be parallel to the wall in front of you (figure 1.28).
- ▶ Reverse the movement, and return to your head and pelvis to the starting position.
- ▶ Repeat 8 times.

Sensing

The key here is to sense the pelvis and head movements at the same time without tensing the muscles at the top of the neck. Your pelvis and head are both part of one movement, which is the lengthening of your entire spine in both directions. This exercise involves exaggerating the backward pull of the neck to break the habit of carrying it too far forward. At the end of the exercise, stop making any effort to pull your head backward. Find a comfortable place to carry it, so it feels like it is balancing on top of your neck with little effort.

8. Seated Wave

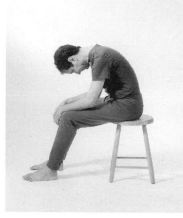

Fig. 1.29

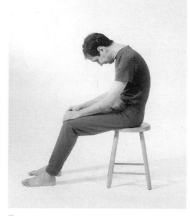

Fig. 1.30

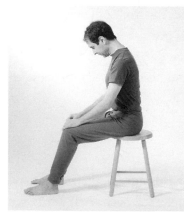

Fig. 1.31

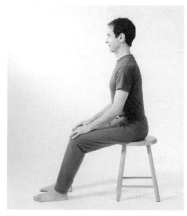

Fig. 1.32

Prerequisite
Explorations 1–6

Objective
To learn how to carry the whole spine naturally.

Position
- Sit forward on a chair or stool, with your chest caved in and your head dropped down. Relax your back muscles completely. Your hands can relax in your lap or between your knees (figure 1.29).
- As you exhale, press your feet into the ground to tilt your pelvis backward. Keep your back rounded and your head down (figure 1.30).
- When the weight on your pelvis has rolled behind your sit bones, reverse the direction of your pelvis as you inhale. Make this a continuous movement, so the transition from backward to forward is smooth. As your pelvis now tilts forward, simultaneously begin to raise your head (figure 1.31).
- Continue tilting your pelvis forward until you are sitting on the front of your sit bones. Your chest and head will be in a fully upright position (figure 1.32). Stay there for a few seconds, long enough to be aware of how you are carrying yourself.
- Return to the starting position, and repeat the backward and forward motion 8 times.

Sensing
This exercise builds on the previous exercises, adding the smooth transition between the backward and forward pelvic tilt. The result is a wave-like movement from your pelvis up to your head. When your pelvis tilts forward in this exercise, feel or imagine a wave moving up your spine from your pelvis to your head. It is similar to the motion of a young plant unfurling upward as it grows. Whether you sense it as a wave or as an inner lengthening of your spine, this movement will gently teach you how to carry your spine naturally.

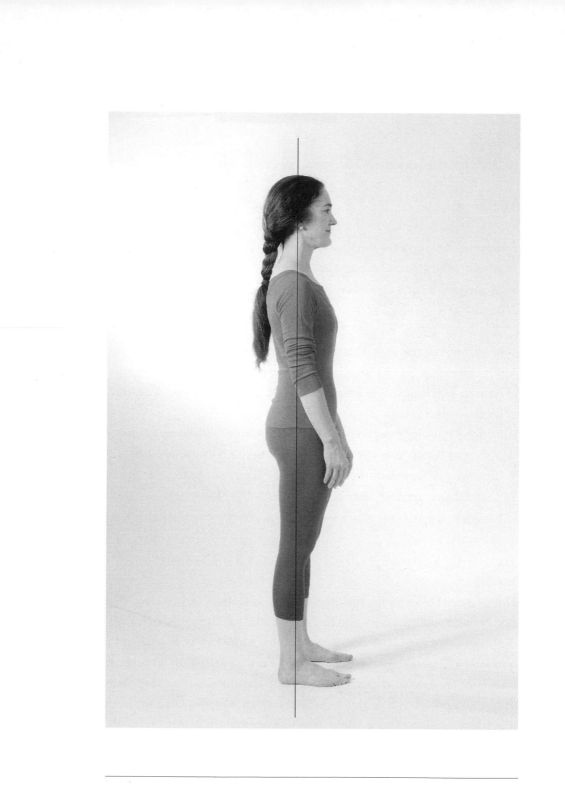

2 Standing

FROM THE MOMENT you were born, you had a relationship with the ground. The earth is your constant companion.

Learning to move and walk involves negotiating with gravity. If you watch a four-month old baby lying on her chest, you can see that much of what she is doing is trying to move part of her body upward or forward. She has a constant relationship with gravity, and her efforts to move develop her muscles and nerves so she will eventually be able to stand. When she does, her head will be far away from her feet, yet she will still be in a relationship with the earth.

I often hear people say that standing involves fighting gravity, suggesting that gravity is something we must override. But gravity is too strong to be conquered, and our bodies know it. We have evolved to use bones, muscles, and connective tissue for leverage, which makes movement in the field of gravity much easier. Our bodies are made to have a cooperative relationship with the ground.

Sometimes, of course, this is not how it feels. This was illustrated by a cartoon I once saw that pictured an alarm clock ringing and a guy struggling to pull himself out of bed, with the caption "Gravity is particularly strong this morning."

GRAVITY AND YOU

Someone who stands with good carriage is not working as hard as someone who stands with poor carriage. If standing is hard work, then gravity feels like an opponent. The body needs to be carried with natural alignment to move easily. "Natural alignment" means in accord with its design, which includes both physics and psychology. So, if we are made to use gravity as a partner, how do we end up with unnatural alignment?

Since the body, mind, and psyche are not separate, how we stand is the result of a lifetime of bodily and psychological influences, such as injuries, emotional conditions, thought patterns, culture, occupations, and physical training. These influences lead to habits and postures that become our "default setting" for standing alignment. If we identify and improve the default setting, we can change our habitually poor standing carriage.

The majority of people I work with have carriage, alignment, or posture problems that are reversible, meaning they can be corrected. Even if you have a genuine structural problem that is not reversible, such as adolescent-onset scoliosis or a true leg-length difference, your movement patterns can be improved, which will improve the movement functioning of your body.

You can begin to change how you use your body by turning your view of gravity upside down. Rather than imagining it only as something that pulls you down, try seeing it as something that also pushes up into your body. When you are standing, the earth is pressing into your feet as much as your feet are pressing into the earth. In physics, this is known as the *ground reactive force*. Paradoxically, the more you feel the force pressing up into your bones, the more your body will relax and feel rooted in the ground. Imagine an upward force traveling through your bones from your feet to your head, guiding the way your bones are positioned. The following exploration will help you.

⹀ Exploration 7

- Stand up and look down at one of your ankles. Notice the two round, prominent bones, one on the inside and one on the outside. These are known as the *medial* and *lateral malleolus*, respectively, which are at the bottom of the two lower leg bones, the *tibia* and *fibula*. Between these ankle protrusions is roughly where the weight of your lower leg balances on top of your foot when you are standing.

- Keeping standing with your feet parallel. Place a round dowel or pencil under both feet so that it presses up into the area at the very back of your arches, just in front of your heels. This will be directly below the medial and lateral malleoli on each foot.

- Focus your attention on the places where you feel the dowel pressing into your feet. If you could line up the rest of your body above those two points, you would have good alignment. Imagine a force moving up from the ground just beneath the dowel and pressing upward through your legs, pelvis, spine, and head. Along the way, this force is moving your bones upward so they are hovering directly above the dowel.

- Step away from the dowel and continue standing. Remember the feeling of where the dowel pressed into your feet as a reference point for where your legs should balance. Relax your ankles—make no particular effort to use your calf muscles.

- Let your entire body sway slightly back and forth, like a tree swaying in the wind. Regardless of which direction you move, keep your weight equally distributed over your feet, as if they were glued to the ground.

- Stop swaying and again find the balance point of your legs on top of your feet. Do your ankles and back feel more relaxed than usual?

The Central Vertical Axis

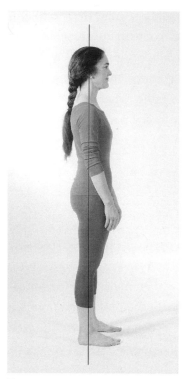

Fig. 2.1

Good standing alignment means your bones are balanced on top of one another. In this case, your bones do as much of the work as possible, while your muscles do the least amount possible. Your hip joints should be directly over your ankles and your upper body directly over your pelvis. You can imagine a vertical line passing through the middle of your body, roughly between your ears, hip joints, and ankles. This line is called your central vertical axis, or your axis of gravity (figure 2.1). It is not necessary to know precisely where the central axis passes, but it is helpful to have a general idea of how the major body parts can line up on top of one another.

The Pelvis

As mentioned in Chapter 1, the pelvis has a left side and a right side. The base of the spine (called the sacrum) is between the two sides of the pelvis and is described in the next section of this chapter.

The hip joints (see figure 1.1) are the two ball-and-socket joints where the pelvis connects to the tops of the legs. The pelvis is not stationary when you are standing; it is continuously balancing on top of your legs. For example, if you were attempting to balance on a ball, you would stand on top of it, not on the back or front. In the same way, the hip sockets of your pelvis are meant to be perched at the top of the femoral heads when you stand. This is the neutral tilt position for the pelvis when standing. Conversely, if you stand with your pelvis tilted too far forward or backward or if it is shifted off center (which will be described shortly), you are no longer balancing on the top of the femoral heads. When this happens, muscles somewhere in your body will tense to help you keep your balance.

Consequently, the two movements most relevant to standing are (1) *tilting* the pelvis forward and backward, and (2) *shifting* the pelvis forward and backward. When you read the descriptions of pelvic tilting and pelvic shifting, visualize each one. People often confuse these two terms, so if it is necessary, stand up and exaggerate the motions so you can feel the difference between tilting and shifting. Doing this will help you understand the explanations of standing alignment that come later.

Another alignment condition is symmetry between the left and right sides of the pelvis. If the two sides are not mirror images, they are said to be asymmetrical. There are many possibilities for asymmetry between the two sides of the pelvis, given the many ways each side is able to rotate, tilt, and turn. Pelvis asymmetry is usually not a problem for good carriage and is not directly addressed by the exercises in this book. Our bodies can give us tremendous leeway for mechanical imperfection. Many people I've worked with have reduced their pain by improving their muscle tone, even though their asymmetry did not visibly change.

Pelvic Tilt

The starting point for improving your standing alignment is to investigate how your pelvis is tilted. To get a sense of this, imagine that your pelvis is a bucket full of water, where the rim of the bucket roughly coincides with the waistband of your pants. If the top of the bucket (the pelvis) is tilted forward, the water pours out the front; if it is tilted backward, the water pours out the back. This analogy is not perfect, because the structure of the pelvis is not much like a bucket; it is more like an upright ring balanced on top of the leg bones. Nonetheless, I find that the bucket analogy is the most helpful way to give people an accurate sense of how the pelvis moves on the hip joints.

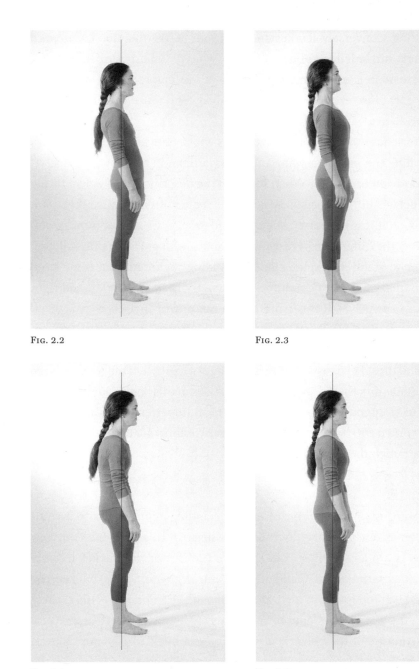

Fɪɢ. 2.2

Fɪɢ. 2.3

Fɪɢ. 2.4

Fɪɢ. 2.5

Recall from Chapter 1 that the neutral tilt position of the pelvis is the one that provides the most support for the spinal curve and the carriage of the head. In standing, you can think of it as the pelvic position that allows your bones to do as much work as possible and your muscles to do as little possible. It is important to remember that neutral pelvic tilt does *not* mean the rim of the imaginary bucket is level with the ground. Neutral tilt is when the pelvis is tilted a little bit forward. One way to find your neutral pelvic tilt in standing is to identify it first when you are sitting (see Exploration 3 in Chapter 1), then practice maintaining the same tilt when you stand up. Exercise 10 in this chapter is designed to help you sense neutral pelvic tilt when standing.

If the pelvis is tilted too far backward or forward when standing (figures 2.2–2.5, compare to figure 2.1), the spine and legs must adapt by modifying their alignment. In the explorations and exercises in Chapter 1, you could feel that tilting your pelvis backward decreases (flattens or reverses) the natural lumbar curve, while tilting your pelvis forward increases the lumbar curve. As for your legs, an excessive backward tilt encourages outward (lateral) rotation, while an excessive forward tilt encourages inward (medial) rotation. This also affects walking, because ideally the feet should point straight ahead, not turn outward or inward. The most common pelvic tilt I see in both sitting and standing is tilted too far backward. This is sometimes mistaken for good posture.

Exploration 8

- Stand with your feet parallel to each other. Press your fingers into the top of your pubic bone, in the center of your pelvis. Then move your fingers horizontally to the left and right, so they are pressing about halfway between your pubic bone and each side of your pelvis. This is approximately where your hip joints are located. These are the hinges that close and open when you squat and stand up.

- Imagine that your pelvis is a bucket and the waistband of your pants is the rim of the bucket. While pressing your fingers into the front of each hip joint, slowly bend your hip hinges while also bending your knees. Feel how your hip joints fold where your fingers are pressing in. As you bend, intentionally tilt your pelvis forward; this means that the water in the bucket would be spilling over the front rim. Notice that the farther forward your pelvis tilts, the greater the folding in your hip joints. Squat down only as far as you feel comfortable, keeping the entire sole of each foot on the ground.

- Press the soles of your feet into the ground and use your legs to return to a standing position. Use your fingertips to feel how your hip hinges are now opening.

- Repeat this small squatting and standing motion at least 10 times. When you begin to bend from the standing position, make sure you initiate the movement by bending at the hip joints and then feel how the rest of your body follows.

- Return to a standing position. Remember the feeling of *where* your hip joints folded and your pelvis tilted. Without bending your knees, find the degree of pelvic tilt that makes you feel that your pelvis is balancing on top of your leg bones. Remain here for a minute to sense how this may differ from your usual standing alignment.

Pelvic Shift

I use the term pelvic shift to describe how the pelvis as a whole can be shifted in front of or behind the central vertical axis. It can happen in the standing position, but it is not relevant to sitting. Shift is easy to see when you observe someone from the side (figures 2.6 through 2.8). Shifting is a different movement than tilting; shifting does not necessarily affect pelvic tilt.

If you imagine a bucket hanging from a long rope, you can picture it swinging forward or backward or hanging straight down. In a similar way, the pelvis can be shifted forward or backward or hang in the mid-

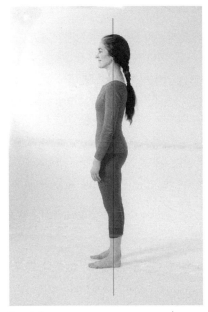

FIG. 2.6

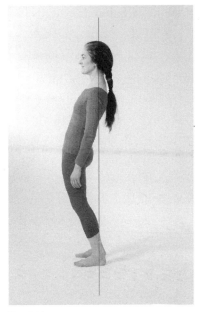

FIG. 2.7

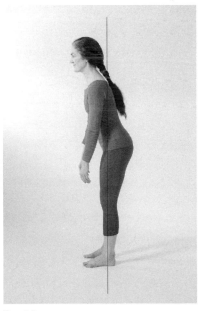

FIG. 2.8

dle when standing. When it is shifted forward or backward, the legs and spine are pulled along with it and away from the central vertical axis. By contrast, when the pelvis is in the middle, the spine and legs are approximately vertical. You can see in figure 2.6 that it is easiest for the chest and head to line up with the rest of the body when the pelvis is not shifted forward or backward.

Standing postures with the pelvis shifted forward are common. When the pelvis shifts forward, it cannot properly support the lumbar spine. In this position, the pelvis leans against ligaments in the front of the hips, much the same way you can lean your pelvis against a counter to help hold yourself up (similar to the alignment shown in figure 2.2). This standing position may feel relaxed to some people because their ligaments are doing most of the work. However, a forward pelvic shift causes some part of the rib cage or upper back to move behind the central vertical axis, which distorts the lumbar curve.

A backward shift is less common. When the pelvis shifts backward, the head or chest will be forced forward to maintain balance (similar to the alignment shown in figure 2.4).

⌐ Exploration 9

- Stand up.

- This time, imagine that your pelvis is a bucket suspended from a long rope. Shift it forward as far as you comfortably can, as if the bucket were swinging forward. Remain in this position as you feel what has happened in the rest of your body. Specifically, has your weight shifted on your feet? Have your knees changed position? Does your lower back feel more compressed? Have your chest and head changed position?

- Return to the starting position. Next, shift your pelvis backward (from a side view, it would appear to be farther back than your ankles). Just as you did in the previous step, notice what has happened in the rest of your body.

- Return to standing normally. Press your fingers into the sides of your pelvis at the level of your pubic bone. Imagine a horizontal line passing through your pelvis between your fingers. By shifting and tilting your pelvis minutely forward and backward, position it so that the imaginary line is directly above the balance point of your feet (recall Exploration 6). This will place you midway between a forward and backward shift. Remain here for a minute to sense how this may differ from your usual standing alignment.

The Spine

The spine is one long structure with many parts that span from the tail-bone to the base of the head (figure 2.9). Each unique spinal bone is a vertebra (the plural is vertebrae). Anatomists divide the thirty-three vertebrae of the spine into four sections, each characterized by either a concave or convex curve. These sections are the sacrum and coccyx, the lumbar spine, the thoracic spine, and the cervical spine. Naming these divisions help us understand the details of the structure, but keep

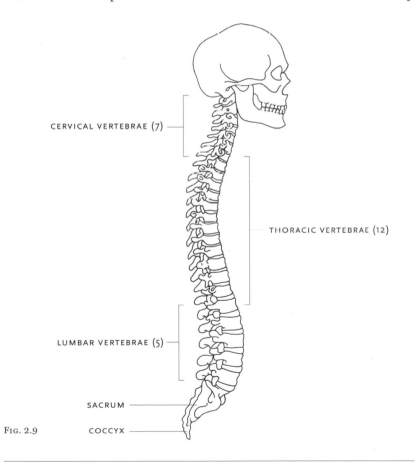

CERVICAL VERTEBRAE (7)

THORACIC VERTEBRAE (12)

LUMBAR VERTEBRAE (5)

SACRUM

Fig. 2.9   COCCYX

in mind that the spine functions as one whole entity, not four separate pieces.

The Sacrum and Coccyx

The sacrum and coccyx (tailbone) are at the base of the spine between the right and left ilium bones of the pelvis. The sacrum is made of five vertebrae that are fused into one triangular-shaped bone. The coccyx, which is below the sacrum, is made of three to five small bones fused into one. The sacrum is in the spine, but because it is sandwiched between the ilium bones, it can also be viewed as part of the pelvic girdle. The sacrum and coccyx have a convex curve when viewed from behind. Because the remainder of the spine rests on top of the sacrum, its alignment affects the carriage of all the vertebrae.

The Lumbar Spine

The five bones of the lumbar spine are commonly called the lower back. The bottom lumbar vertebra rests on top of the sacrum. Since the top of the sacrum is tilted forward, the front of the bottom lumbar vertebra is tilted downward. This results in the natural lumbar curve, which is concave when viewed from behind.

Problems can arise in the lumbar spine when its curve is flattened because of habitually poor carriage. These problems include damaged spinal discs, damaged joints, and hardened spinal muscles.

The Thoracic Spine

The thoracic section of the spine is made up of twelve vertebrae. These vertebrae are where the twelve ribs attach to the spine. The thoracic spine is mildly convex when viewed from behind.

When the pelvis is shifted forward, the rib cage is often shifted backward, behind the central vertical axis (see figure 2.2). When this happens, the shoulders are typically rounded inward and the head and neck project forward. I refer to this as "collapsed posture," because the waist appears to be deflated and collapsed.

The Cervical Spine

The cervical spine is the neck, which has seven vertebrae. Similar to the lumbar spine, the cervical spine has a concave curve when viewed from behind. The head balances on top of the cervical spine.

As mentioned earlier, when the thoracic spine is either too curved and/or shifted behind the central vertical axis, the head and neck typically project forward. When the neck is slanted forward, the muscles in the back of the neck are constantly strained. The neck needs to be fairly upright to function properly, because then the weight of the head is balanced on top of the spine. The better this balance, the less work the neck muscles need to do.

Even the word *neck* can contribute to the misperception that the top seven vertebrae are separate from the rest of the spine. Despite how it may appear, your neck is not something that comes out of your shoulders; it is the top of something that comes out of your pelvis. A mime artist knows this, because to mimic a giraffe, he will bend his entire spine forward from the hip joints, as if the neck begins in the pelvis, to give the impression of a very long neck. Imagine that your neck begins in the middle of your pelvis and notice how your carriage changes.

When there is constant tension in the neck muscles, the head cannot move freely. The tension pulls the head down in either the back or the front. The remainder of the body adjusts to this downward pull on the head by increasing muscle tension throughout the limbs and torso. Surprising as it may sound, the force of gravity, combined with good carriage of the pelvis and spine, causes the head to lift because the neck is free of unnecessary tension.

THE FEET

Feet are hands made for standing. Feet and hands have many things in common. The two we will look at are (1) a grasping action and (2) an arch.

The Grasping Action of the Foot

The feet and hands work with a similar grasping action. It will be easier for you to feel this action in your hands, so let's use them as a way to familiarize you with the same action in your feet. When you grasp something, such as an apple, with your hand, your thumb and fingers move toward each other as your palm folds. Slowly open and close one of your hands right now; observe how the thumb moves toward the other four fingers and vice versa. Your hand is made to hold things. The curved lines on your palm are the result of grasping.

Feet have a natural grasping action too; they are made to grasp the ground. You can feel this while walking barefoot through soft sand at the beach. Unfortunately, many people have lost their kinesthetic sense of this grasping action. As a result, their feet are not responsive to the surfaces they stand on. Instead of behaving like a pair of hands at the ends of the legs, their feet are like rigid pedestals or lifeless flippers. Happily, you can improve the responsiveness of your feet by practicing the foot exercises in this book.

The Arch of the Foot

The arch of the foot is both a structure and an action, and both are important. The bones, ligaments, and muscles of your foot form an arch in the bottom. Technically, the arch of the foot is three different arches. Two are lengthwise: one from the heel toward the first three toes, and the other

Fig. 2.10

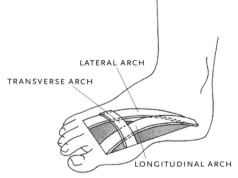

LATERAL ARCH

TRANSVERSE ARCH

LONGITUDINAL ARCH

from the heel toward the fourth and fifth toe. The third arch is perpendicular to the other two, across the middle of the foot. We will refer only to "the arch of the foot," as if the three are one whole arch (figure 2.10).

If you cannot sense the arch in each foot, it may be easier to feel the arch of your hand. Try this. Place your forearm and palm down on a table; relax your muscles. Slowly move your four fingers toward your thumb, keeping your thumb stationary. Feel and see how your palm arches up. Now move your fingers away from your thumb and notice that the arch goes down—but not all the way. Your hand will not naturally lie perfectly flat on the table. To flatten the arch completely, you must either tighten your hand muscles or place a weight on top of your hand.

You can feel the arches in your feet as well. Explorations 10 and 13 and Exercises 14, 15, and 21 will help you do this. The arch acts as a spring, a shock absorber for the foot. It allows the foot to yield to the ground with each step. This makes the rest of the body more comfortable when standing and walking.

In standing and walking, the arch is influenced by an imaginary line in the foot I call the *weight-bearing line*. Look at figure 2.11, the sole of the foot, and notice the position of the *calcaneus* (heel bone). See how it is angled inward, not parallel to the toes. The direction of the

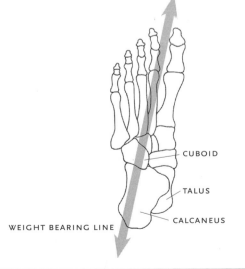

Fig. 2.11

CUBOID

TALUS

CALCANEUS

WEIGHT BEARING LINE

calcaneus shows where the weight of the body wants to travel along the foot when walking. Body weight is carried along this imaginary line, which runs diagonally from the outside half of the calcaneus toward the space between the first and second toe.

In Exploration 7, you placed a dowel under the back of your arch, which is roughly where the weight of your leg balances on top of your foot. It is also the area of your foot that first touches the ground when you are walking barefoot. The outside of the foot is made to bear more weight than the inside. The *cuboid* bone and outside of the calcaneus are solidly on the ground, while the arch keeps most of the inside bones off the ground. The arch causes body weight to flow toward the outside of each foot.

The feet are mobile platforms on which the lower legs balance. These platforms will be level if the feet have a natural arch and are standing on an even surface. Your feet and ankles are remarkably capable of adjusting to uneven ground by tilting and turning. When you stand on a bumpy surface, the platforms of your feet shift constantly, and your body adjusts accordingly.

When the arch is insufficient, the platform of the foot slants inward, causing the lower leg and knee to tilt inward as well. Just as when you stand on uneven ground, the rest of your body compensates for this tilted base of support; the resulting inward tilt of the lower leg can create a chain of compensations that affect your knee, hip, and lower back.

Many of my clients arrive with orthotic arch supports in their shoes. If they have experienced definite, lasting pain relief from these supports, I generally suggest they continue to use them. Otherwise, it is best to avoid anything that interferes with the natural action of your feet, whether it is the shoe itself or an orthotic support. Artificial arch supports will not strengthen the responsiveness of your feet or teach your feet how to have an arch. If your feet tire easily, put special emphasis on the foot exercises in this book. If possible, walk barefoot for a few minutes each day, implementing what you have learned from the exercises. Walking barefoot gives your feet a chance to respond naturally to the ground.

Many people label their feet *pronated*, or *flat*, thinking their arches are like hopelessly collapsed buildings. This is a mistake. Your arch doesn't need to be perfect looking in order to function properly. What matters most is how your feet sense the ground.

RELAXED ANKLES

The ankle is the joint where the lower leg balances on top of the foot. The foot bones are like a strategically arranged pile of stones; the stone on the top of the pile is called the talus bone. The weight of the leg rests on the talus, and from there, it spreads throughout the foot. The lower leg muscles move the ankle joint.

The foot hangs freely at the end of the leg, which you can feel if you lift your foot with your ankle relaxed. Similarly, when standing, your lower leg moves freely on top of your foot. If your pelvis is aligned with the central vertical axis and you relax your ankle muscles, your legs will easily balance on top of your feet. Freedom of ankle movement is important for relaxing the rest of the body, all the way up to the neck.

Ankle movement is limited when the calf or foot muscles are too tense when standing. Many people unconsciously tense their lower leg muscles, holding their ankles in a fixed position, which makes balance more difficult. To adjust, the neck muscles automatically tighten to hold the head in a fixed position. The next exploration will increase your sense of natural ankle movement.

⬄ Exploration 10

- Lie on your back with your legs straight.

- Turn both feet so the soles face each other (inversion). As you do, slide your heels toward each other and rotate your legs so your kneecaps move away from each other (lateral rotation). Your pelvis may naturally want to tilt backward as you do this, which is fine.

- Now turn both feet so the soles face away from each other (eversion). As you do, slide your heels away from each other and rotate your legs so your kneecaps move toward each other (medial rotation). Flex your ankles as if you are trying to pull your outside toes toward your ears. Your pelvis may naturally want to tilt forward as you do this, which is fine.

- Alternate between these two movements 12 times. Notice how your foot twists as you turn your ankles and rotate your legs. This motion is an excellent way to relax your ankles. Along with Exercises 15 and 16, this exploration is helpful in gaining a better sense of the action of your arches.

THREE FREQUENTLY ASKED QUESTIONS ABOUT STANDING

Below are three questions that people commonly ask me. These questions are a result of contrasting information that is widely available about muscle use and alignment.

What about My Abdominal Muscles?

Many people get a genuine feeling of well-being from exercising their abdominal muscles. As long as you can apply the alignment principles described in this book, you can do any kind of exercise you want. There is no particular need, though, to do lengthy abdominal strengthening routines to be able to sit, stand, and walk with good carriage. The explorations and exercises in this book are sufficient to give you the abdominal muscle tone you need for that.

It is important to relax any unnecessary muscle tension in your abdomen. Tense *rectus abdominal* muscles interfere with tilting your pelvis forward and sometimes also pull the front of your rib cage down too far. Some people tense these muscles in an attempt to tuck their pelvis under, because they were taught it was good for their back or that it was the model of good posture (see figure 2.5). I do not recommend this for two reasons. First, most people I see already stand with their pelvis tilted too far back. Second, there is no need to hold the pelvis in any particular position. It will balance properly on top of the legs if it is tilted the right way.

Abdominal muscle tone is important because these muscles help support the trunk of the body (see *Muscular Retraining for Pain-Free Living*, pages 87–89). Among other things, good muscle tone in the *transverse* and *oblique abdominals* helps keep the lumbar spine from being compressed, and good tone in the *rectus abdominals* prevents overextension of the back. Moderately engaging the abdominal muscles in an exercise can encourage the lower back muscles to relax, such as in Exercises 1 and 14. This explains why some people experience a relief from lower back pain after doing abdominal exercises. There are many different kinds of useful exercises for the abdomen.

The transverse abdominals lift the rib cage and keep it in a level position. If these muscles do not have enough tone, the chest will sink down. The next exploration will help you feel the important role of the transverse abdominals in the alignment of your upper body, especially in correcting collapsed posture. (See *Muscular Retraining for Pain-Free Living*, pages 92–94, to learn more about this.)

⩵ Exploration 11

- Sit on a stool facing a wall. Move your knees apart as far as is comfortable and touch your toes to the wall. Place your fingertips on the wall just above your head. Imagine that you are holding a ball under each hand so that your palms and fingers are rounded.

- Press all of your fingertips into the wall firmly as you slowly walk your fingers up the wall. Relax your neck and shoulder muscles as much as you can. Keep pressing your fingertips into the wall. As your hands go higher, you will feel your abdominal muscles engage.

These are the transverse abdominals, which are lifting your rib cage to help your arms reach higher. Continue to walk your fingers upward until your arms are extended.

- Keeping the same abdominal muscles engaged, bring your arms down to your side. Notice how your sitting alignment has changed. Repeat the same process once or twice, until you can clearly feel the action of the transverse abdominals in lifting your rib cage.

- Stand up while you try to keep the same abdominal muscles lightly engaged. If you lose the feeling of engagement in those muscles, do the same finger-climbing movement against the wall—this time in the standing position.

- Notice if you are standing differently when these muscles are lightly engaged. Walk around for a minute to feel this as well. If you tend toward a collapsed posture, you will benefit from reinforcing this feeling of a longer waist until it becomes second nature. When the tone of your transverse abdominals is good and your pelvis is in neutral alignment, the subtle lifting of your rib cage is automatic.

Is My Lower Back Too Curved?

I have worked with many people who have been told by a health practitioner that their lower back is "too curved." To remedy this, they make a conscious effort to tilt their pelvis backward. Some have told me they experienced lower back relief for a while from this tilt. How is that possible? For someone with collapsed posture, intentionally tilting the pelvis backward can relieve the compressed lower back muscles. In the long run, though, this involves an unnecessary use of the abdominal muscles, potentially flattening the lumbar curve and restricting the mobility of the pelvis. More relief can be had, with less effort and no harmful side effects, by tilting the pelvis forward so it is balanced correctly over the legs.

When I begin working with these people, I suggest that they stop trying to tilt their pelvis backward and observe what happens when they apply the alignment principles I teach them. In nearly all cases, their lumbar curve turns out to be fine.

Most of the people who have misidentified their lumbar spine as being too curved usually stand with their pelvis shifted forward, which can give a false impression of too much curvature (see figure 2.2). In actuality, the curve of the lower back is being compressed because the chest is shifted backward, behind the pelvis. The solution is to shift (not tilt) the pelvis back to the central vertical axis so it balances over the top of the legs, which automatically brings the chest forward. When this happens, the lumbar spine is no longer compressed, so it returns to its normal length and curve. The spine was okay all along, but it had been in a position that didn't allow for its natural long arc.

I often use Exercise 9 to help people find their natural lumbar curve when standing. After a few minutes of this exercise, their lumbar spine is typically more curved than usual. When I tell them they are now standing with a natural curve, they commonly reply, "It feels like my butt is sticking out." I then have them look in a full-length mirror to see that the lumbar curve is not actually exaggerated, even though it feels that way. Within a week or two of practicing the exercise, they typically tell me that the new pelvis and lumbar position now feels normal and their back is more relaxed.

Do I Need to Pull My Shoulders Back So I Don't Slouch?
Not really. If your shoulders are slumped forward and your chest is sunken, your head is forced forward and the space into which your lungs can expand is decreased. This posture is caused by the way you carry your thoracic spine, which is too rounded. This causes your chest to cave in and your entire shoulder girdle to move forward (see figure 2.4).

In this situation, your shoulders appear to be too far forward, so pulling them back with your upper back muscles may appear to be the solution. It does temporarily solve the rounded shoulders problem, but it does not change its fundamental cause, which is a too-curved thoracic spine.

If you want to stop slouching, you first need to change the way you carry your pelvis and lumbar spine. When they are well aligned, they will provide the base for a natural thoracic curve. Your chest will feel more open, so it will be easier to breathe fully. With your chest open, you can just relax your shoulders and let your arms hang at your sides. There is no need to pull your shoulders back. Imagine that your shoulder girdle is hanging from your head like a cape. If you cannot sense how the lumbar curve helps to keep your chest upright, then review the exercises in Chapter 1.

If you have been narrowing the front of your chest and rounding your shoulders for years, you may benefit from exercises that widen your chest. A narrowed chest usually involves tension and kinesthetic dysfunction of the chest and/or upper back muscles that attach to the shoulder blades. In this case, the shortened chest muscles may need extra help to relax and return to their normal length. Exercises that engage the upper back muscles to rotate the arms backward and/or pull the shoulder blades downward help to address this (for examples, see *Muscular Retraining for Pain-Free Living*, pages 174–176).

After you finish practicing chest-opening exercises, stop pulling your shoulders back and relax. Remind yourself that the width from shoulder to shoulder across the top of your chest is the same as the width from shoulder to shoulder across the top of your upper back. If you are not convinced, you can confirm it with a tape measure.

BENDING DOWN

The following exploration focuses on different stages of bending at the hip joints. The idea is to find a functional way to bend toward the ground and retain some sense of your lumbar curve. If you need to reach down for a prolonged time, such as to pull weeds in your garden, this will be a more comfortable position than just hanging over from your waist.

⊒ Exploration 12

- Get on your hands and knees, with your hands directly below your shoulders as in Part One of Exercise 7. Relax your lower back, abdominal, chest, and shoulder muscles. In this position, gravity will encourage you to sense your lumbar curve without any tension in your lower back. Remain in this position until you can feel the relaxed curve in your lumbar spine.

- Stand up and place your hands on a table that is about waist-height. Bend your knees a little. Remember the way your lower back curved inward when you were on your knees; relax your back so that it feels the same way, even though you are now standing up. You will be bending at the hip joints. Stay in this position for 30 seconds.

- Rest your arms and head on the table while keeping your knees bent. You will be bending more fully at the hip joints than before. Remember the way your lower back curved inward in the first two positions; relax your back so it feels the same way in this new position. Remain here for 30 seconds.

- Take your arms and head off the table and let them hang freely toward the floor. Keep your knees bent a little. Your hip joint hinges are folded closed now, like a book that is closed. The front of your pelvis should nearly touch the fronts of your thighs. Remember the way your lower back curved inward in the previous three positions, and try to achieve the same curve in this position. Imagine you are looking for something on the ground and are also trying to reach the ground in a way that is comfortable for your back. In this position, with your pelvis tilted forward and your lower back curved inward, your legs do most of the work. Your legs are bent only enough to allow your pelvis to tilt forward easily, not so much that they will tire quickly. Remain in this position for 30 seconds, then stand up. Remember how it feels and use it when you need to bend down for extended periods of time.

KEY POINTS FOR STANDING

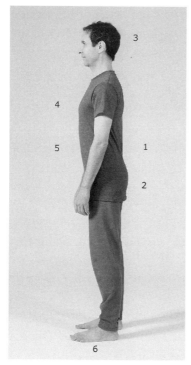

FIG. 2.12

1. The lumbar spine is naturally curved: Explorations 3 and 8; Exercises 8, 9, and 17

2. The pelvis is directly below the upper body: Explorations 7 and 9; Exercise 10

3. The head is directly over the upper body: Explorations 7 and 9; Exercises 7, 8, 10, and 16

4. The chest is open, and the shoulders are relaxed: Explorations 1–4; Exercises 6–8 and 16

5. The core muscles support the upper body: Explorations 7 and 11; Exercises 10–13

6. Body weight is centered over the balance point of the feet, and the arches support the feet: Explorations 7 and 10; Exercises 10, 14, and 15

KEY POINTS FOR BENDING AT THE HIPS

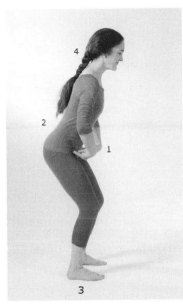

FIG. 2.13

1. Bending down begins at the hinges of the hip joints: Explorations 8 and 12; Exercises 3, 9, and 12

2. The pelvis tilts forward as the hips bend, and the natural lumbar curve is preserved: Explorations 2 and 5; Exercises 9 and 17

3. Body weight is distributed evenly over the feet, including the heels: Explorations 7 and 10; Exercise 10

4. The neck is in line with the rest of the spine: Explorations 7 and 12; Exercises 10 and 16

STANDING EXERCISES

More balance is involved in standing than in sitting, because unlike a chair, your legs need to remain flexible while continuing to support your body. Standing is a balancing act. What you learned from the Chapter 1 exercises about carrying your pelvis, spine, and head is a foundation for standing.

9. STANDING MINI SQUAT

Prerequisites
Explorations 4, 5, 8, and 12

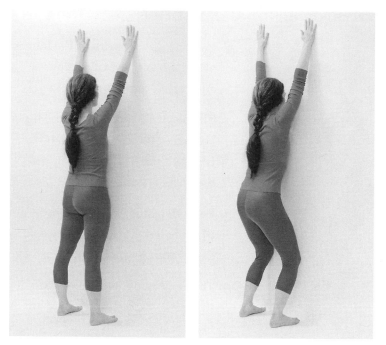

FIG. 2.14 FIG. 2.15

Objective

To sense the neutral pelvic tilt and lumbar curve in a standing position.

Position

- ▶ Face a wall, with your feet about four inches from it, your arms outstretched over your head, and your palms on the wall (figure 2.14).
- ▶ Relax your abdominal muscles so that the front of your pelvis tilts forward; this begins to fold your hip joints. Continue to bend your hips and knees so that your lower body drops down a few inches, but keep your hands in place (figure 2.15). *Do not tense your lower back muscles.* You will feel a definite inward curve in your lower back, which is the point. Stay in this position for 10 to 20 seconds.
- ▶ Next, slowly straighten your knees, doing your best to keep your pelvis tilted forward and your abdominal muscles relaxed. Again, do not tense your lower back muscles; maintain the same lumbar curve.

When your legs are fully straight, you may feel that the curve in your lumbar spine is greater than usual.

▸ Repeat the same process 3 times. Afterward, use this pelvic and spinal position when standing and walking.

Sensing

Feel how bending at your hip joints begins with tilting your pelvis forward. Notice that your lower abdominal muscles need to relax for you to do this without tensing your back muscles. Imagine that you are hanging from a bar that is just low enough for your feet touch the ground. This may give you a feeling of greater length between your chest and pubic bone, which means your lower back has a renewed curve. Also, there is no need to shift your pelvis backward to get your hips to bend. If your back gets tired while you do this exercise, then it is working too hard. Try pressing your feet into the floor while you are in the squatting position.

10. WALL PLANK

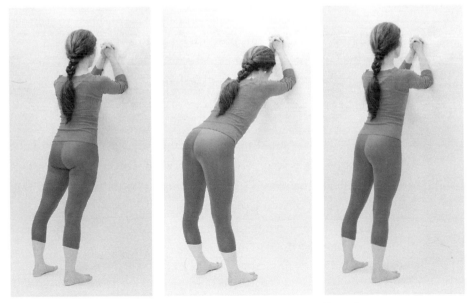

FIG. 2.16   FIG. 2.17   FIG.2.18

Prerequisites
Explorations 7–12

Objective
To sense how the abdominal muscles keep the rib cage aligned with the central vertical axis.

Position
▸ Stand facing a wall, with your feet parallel to each other and about three feet from the wall. Lean forward and place your forearms against the wall at shoulder-level (figure 2.16). Look directly in front of you.

▸ Slowly shift your pelvis backward, placing as much weight on your heels as possible. As you shift your pelvis backward, tilt it slightly forward. Keep your lower back relaxed and curved inward. Stop in the position where you feel the most weight on your heels (figure 2.17).

▸ Next, very slowly *shift* your pelvis forward while keeping the same amount of pressure on your heels. Keep your pelvis tilted forward—do not tilt it backward at all. Keep gradually shifting your pelvis forward until it aligns with your head and feet (figure 2.18). Keep your lower back relaxed. Remain in this position for 10 to 20 seconds.

▸ Repeat the same process 3 times. Afterward, use this carriage in your trunk and head when standing and walking.

Sensing
Sense how your abdominal muscles need to engage for you to keep weight on your heels as your pelvis shifts forward. This is an exaggeration of what the abdominals need to do in a normal standing position. Feel how the entire back of your body, from your head to your heels, lengthens without your pelvis being tilted backward. Also feel how your chest and head are lifted by the combined action of your spine and abdominal muscles.

11. Easy Foot Slide

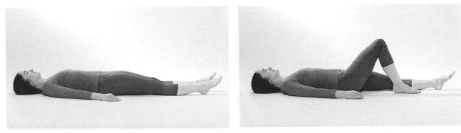

FIG. 2.19   FIG. 2.20

Prerequisite
Exploration 11

Objective
To control the movement of the leg from the hip while keeping the lower leg relaxed. This can be applied directly to walking.

Position
- ▶ Lie on your back with your legs straight, and your arms comfortably on the ground at your sides (figure 2.19).
- ▶ Slowly bend your right knee by sliding your right foot along the floor (figure 2.20). Then straighten your knee by sliding your foot back to the starting position. Continue sliding your foot back and forth.
- ▶ Try to keep your pelvis still and your lower back long throughout the exercise. That is, do not arch your back up and increase your lumbar curve or forcefully press your lower back downward.
- ▶ Perform the movement 8 times with your right leg, then repeat 8 times with your left.

Sensing
Imagine that your femur (thighbone) is a fishing rod. The handle of the rod is at your hip joint; the end of the rod is at your knee. As you slide your foot back and forth, imagine that you are controlling the movement of

your thigh by using the handle, just as you would with a fishing rod. This means you relax the muscles in your lower thigh, knee, and lower leg.

12. Supine Hip Flexor Leg Raise

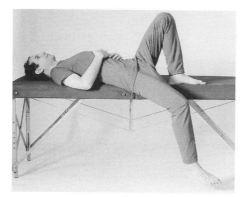
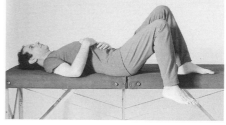

Fig. 2.21 (LEFT)
Fig. 2.22 (ABOVE)

Prerequisite
Exploration 11

Objective
To control the movement of the leg from the hip while keeping the lower leg relaxed. This can be applied directly to walking.

Position
- Lie on your back on top of a table or bed. Lie at an angle, so that your right leg hangs off the edge. Your pelvis and upper body remain on the table. Bend your left knee and place your left foot flat on the table (figure 2.21). If your lower back is uncomfortable in this position, then hold your left knee with both hands and pull it toward your chest.
- Raise your right knee *very slowly*, keeping your lower leg relaxed and dangling from the knee. Whenever you find yourself beginning to straighten your right knee, stop, let the lower leg relax, and then go on. Continue to raise your right leg until it is approximately at the level of the table or bed (figure 2.22).

- Lower your leg *very slowly* in the same fashion. When it is all the way down, relax completely.
- Perform this movement 8 times on your right side and then 8 times on your left.

Sensing

Feel how the control of raising and lower your leg comes from the front of your pelvis and the top of your thigh. Relax the muscles around your knee and lower leg, so your lower leg hangs down from the knee. Keep your pelvis in a neutral position throughout the movement; don't tilt it forward or backward.

13. MODIFIED DOUBLE LEG SLIDE

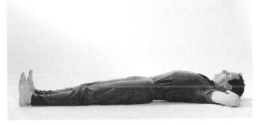

FIG. 2.23

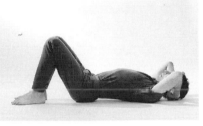

FIG. 2.24

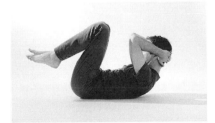

FIG. 2.25

Prerequisite
Exploration 11

Objective

To strengthen the core muscles.

Position

▸ Lie on your back with your legs straight and your legs and feet parallel to each other. Place your hands under the back of your head (figure 2.23).

▸ As you inhale, slowly bend your knees as you slide your feet along the floor. Keep your pelvis in a neutral tilt, so there is a small lumbar curve, during this part of the exercise. Slide your feet until they are flat on the ground with your knees bent (figure 2.24).

▸ Exhale and continue to move your legs in the same direction by raising your feet off the ground. In this phase of the exercise, use your abdominal muscles to roll your pelvis backward and press your lower back into the ground. Simultaneously, use your abdominal muscles and arms to pick up your head (figure 2.25). Point your elbows upward as you use your arms and keep your neck relaxed.

▸ Inhale and bring your head and feet down by gradually relaxing your abdominal muscles. When your feet touch the floor, keep your knees bent.

▸ Exhale as you straighten your knees and slide your feet back to the starting position (figure 2.23).

▸ Repeat this movement 8 times.

Sensing

Feel how the movement of your legs and arms can be relatively relaxed when the abdominal and hip flexor muscles are smoothly engaging and releasing throughout the movement. The more you can control the tension and relaxation in these core muscles the easier it is to relax your limbs.

14. Foot Sweep

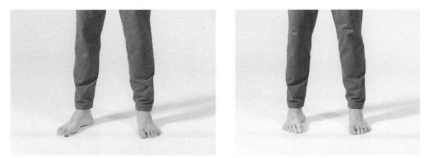

Fig. 2.26   Fig. 2.27

Prerequisite
Exploration 10

Objective
To improve the muscle tone in the arch of the foot.

Position
- ▸ Stand with your feet parallel (figure 2.26). Turn the front of your right foot outward, keeping your heel in place, so that the toes are pointing out to the side.
- ▸ Bring your foot back to parallel by sliding the outside edge of your foot and the tips of your toes against the ground (figure 2.27). As you make this sweeping motion, your arch will increase.
- ▸ Perform this movement 8 times with your right foot, then 8 times with your left.

Sensing
Feel how this effort in your foot raises the arch.

15. Foot Arch

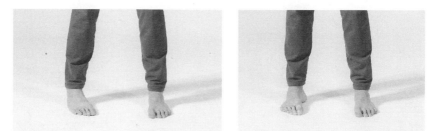

Fig. 2.28   Fig. 2.29

Prerequisite
Exploration 10

Objective
To improve the muscle tone in the arch of the foot.

Position
- Stand with your feet parallel. Turn your right heel outward while keeping your toes in place (figure 2.28). Take your weight off your right heel by lifting it slightly off the ground.
- Grasping the ground with your toes and the ball of your foot, swing your heel back to the parallel position (figure 2.29). As you do this, the grasping action of your foot muscles will cause your foot to twist, lifting your arch. Similar to the previous exercise, the outside edge of your foot remain on the ground as the inside of your foot goes up. Allow your knee to move outward as necessary to let your heel move inward.
- Do 8 repetitions with each foot. If you have very weak feet, it will helpful for you to do several sets of the arch exercises daily.

Sensing
Feel how the muscles in the sole of your foot can move your heel inward. Also, feel how this effort raises the inside of your foot and presses down the outside edge.

16. Prone Neck Rotation with Extension

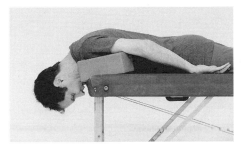

Fig. 2.30

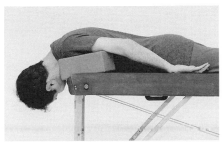

Fig. 2.31

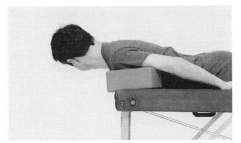

Fig. 2.32

Prerequisites
Explorations 5 and 6

Objective
To free the head from the neck muscles and correct the position of the head on the spine while sitting and standing.

Position

- Lie facedown on a bed or table so that your head hangs completely over the edge; your chin should *not* touch the side of the bed. Place a yoga block or rolled towel under the front of each shoulder and upper arm (figure 2.30).

- To begin, let your head hang freely until the muscles in the back of your neck relax.

- Turn your head slowly right and left as far as you comfortably can (figure 2.31). Keep the muscles in the back of your neck relaxed so that you feel your head is dangling from your neck as it rotates to each side. Turn to each side 6 times.

- Next, turn your head to the right again and hold it in this position as you raise it as high as you comfortably can (figure 2.32). Use the muscles in your lower and upper back and the sides of your neck to help raise your head, *but do not shorten or tighten the muscles at the top of the back of your neck.*

▶ Slowly lower your head in the same fashion, waiting until it is all the way down before turning it back to the middle position. When your head is back at center, check to make certain that the muscles in the back of your neck are relaxed.

▶ Turn your head to the left and repeat the same procedure of raising and lowering it slowly. Repeat for a total of 3 times to each side.

Sensing

Feel that your head is dangling from your neck and that it can turn and lift without bunching up the muscles in the back of your neck. Imagine that your head is leading your neck as it moves—that is, that your head is turning itself and your neck is following.

17. Leg Raise on All Fours

Prerequisite
Exploration 6

Objective
To strengthen the hip and back extensors and increase the kinesthetic sense of the lumbar curve.

Position

▶ Kneel on all fours with your right leg extended straight behind you. Turn your leg out (rotate it laterally) from the hip so the inside of your right foot is against the floor. If this position hurts your wrists, make a fist with each hand so your wrists are not bent. Keep your neck in line with the rest of your spine; look at the floor directly below you (figure 2.33).

▶ As you inhale, slowly raise your right leg so that it is horizontal or higher. As your leg goes up, your pelvis will tilt slightly forward and

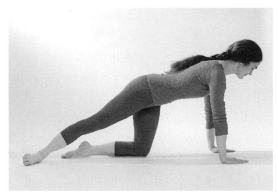

FIG. 2.33

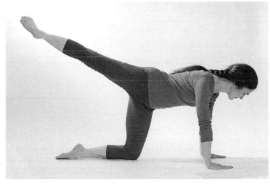

FIG. 2.34

rotate to the right (so the right side of your pelvis is higher than the left).

▸ As you exhale, slowly return your right leg to the starting position.

▸ Do this motion slowly 8 times, then repeat with your left leg.

Sensing

Feel how your lower back muscles work to lift your leg. At the same time, notice how your pelvis tilts forward, so the front of your trunk lengthens from neck to pelvis. You can use this exercise to regain the feeling of a long, gradual lumbar curve. Stand up after doing this exercise to feel how it has affected your alignment.

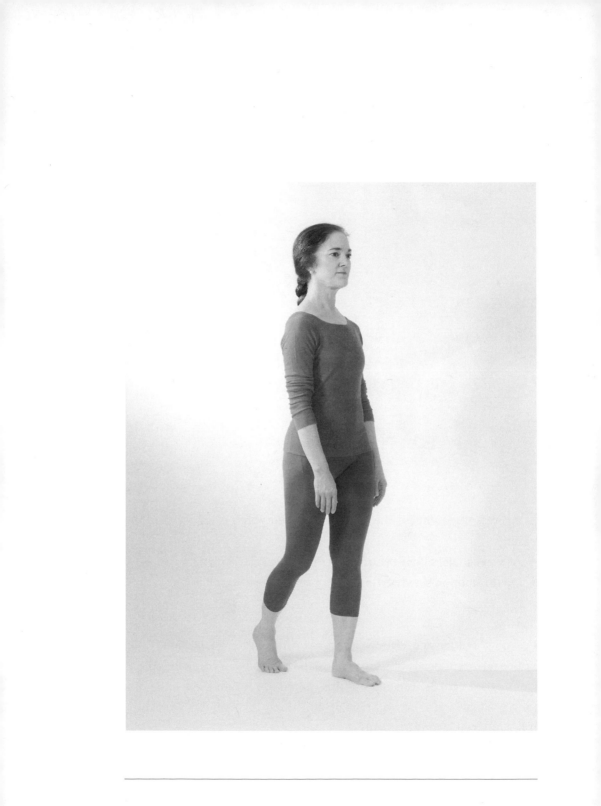

3 Walking

WHEN YOU WALK, you usually only have one foot on the ground at a time, and you are able to pass your entire body weight from one leg to the other without falling to the side. Amazing, but true.

The way you walk has a lot to do with how you stand. So everything I have said about standing also applies to walking. To walk well, you need to have good standing carriage and then move forward while maintaining that carriage. If necessary, review the exercises for standing in Chapter 2.

CONNECTION TO THE EARTH

We all have an existential relationship with the earth that is evident when we consider the ordinary movements involved with standing and walking. One aspect of this relationship is the security that comes from being able to balance and walk without falling. Another aspect is relaxation, which allows us to sense our connection to the earth and to enjoy moving our bodies. Many people end up sacrificing relaxation for security, resulting in muscle tension and poor alignment. There is no need to choose between security and relaxation, because when your alignment is good they reinforce each other.

Security

I sometimes use my hands to help guide an individual client into a new standing position, so he can sense how it feels for his body mass to be centered along the central vertical axis. It is not unusual for the client to say that he feels like he is going to fall over, even though he is more securely balanced than usual. Looking in a mirror will visually convince him that he is balanced, but he may still feel unstable. Like some people, he may find this new position intolerable and immediately shift back to his familiar posture. To become comfortable with an aligned stance, he will need to do the exercises in this book until his kinesthetic sense allows him to recognize how off-center his typical stance is. With this new awareness he can know to feel, from the inside, what good alignment is.

I have found that physical insecurity is behind many people's unusual postures and movement patterns. Like all animals, we are born with an innate sense of how to find balance. When a toddler is learning to stand and walk, her wobbling and occasional falls gradually give her the information she needs to learn how to balance. Her muscle tone develops from the trial and error of walking. But at any age, physical, emotional, or mental distress can reset normal muscle tone, making some muscles too tense and others too slack. When this happens, the muscles cannot respond normally to the sensory-motor system, which is trying to maintain standing balance. The result is literally physical insecurity.

Interestingly, I have found that many people, even some accomplished athletes, are unaware of this insecurity. How can they not sense it? Because they have compensated for it and don't realize they are doing so; they've gotten used to it. At a young age, they adjusted their carriage to deal with physical insecurity by subconsciously tightening certain muscles and accepting the inflexibility that went with it. As a result, their kinesthetic sense was diminished, and they ended up overusing their eyes for balance. This all resulted in dysfunctional movement patterns (see *Muscular Retraining for Pain-Free Living*, pages 31–51).

It is important to realize that your brain is very devoted to preventing you from falling over and hurting yourself. If there is a thought or fear of falling, even if you are not conscious of it, your muscles will become tense. If this happens constantly, you get used to it; it becomes the normal background feeling of having a body. The tension compounds as time passes, resulting in the aches and pains that are mistaken for "getting older."

Relaxation

To regain the natural security of balance, muscle tone throughout the body needs to return to normal. An important part of this is relaxing unnecessary muscle tension. When you are relaxed, you carry yourself with better alignment. You are more likely to feel your connection to the ground, which is a natural source of confidence. The earth is a living presence that supports us in many ways, including helping us to relax.

People who live in urban or high-tech environments need to remind themselves daily that they are on the planet and bound to it by gravity. A simple way to do that is to walk. While you are walking, sense the world around you and use your kinesthetic awareness to sense how your body feels. Feel the ground pressing into your feet and up through your leg bones. If you relax when you walk, you will feel your bones doing most of the work. This will help connect you to the earth.

Interestingly, when it comes to strength, a relaxed muscle is stronger than a tense muscle. Some people find that strength training, such as weight lifting, makes their whole body feel better. If you want to train your muscles to be stronger, first learn how to sense and relax them kinesthetically. Then, you will get better results when you do strengthening exercises and won't hurt yourself. Weight-training instructors have thanked me for my explanations of kinesthesia, relaxation, and muscle tone in *Muscular Retraining for Pain-Free Living*, telling me they've long since realized the importance of these elements in their own work.

WALKING

Humans have been walking for thousands of years. Just as birds are built to fly, we are built to walk. Even though the legs do most of the work, every part of the musculoskeletal system is involved in walking. To illustrate this point, I sometimes tell my clients that if all the kinesthetic and movement exercises I teach were combined into one exercise, the result would be walking. In other words, each exercise involves a particular element, or elements, of walking. Because of this, I can observe someone's gait to find dysfunctional movement patterns throughout his body. Similarly, that person can use walking to correct the movement patterns, muscle tone, and alignment of his entire body.

Because the body, mind, and psyche are not separate, walking involves more than what is called "body mechanics." It reflects the whole person, not just muscles and bones. Your pattern of walking shows not only how you use your body to move, but how you move through your life. Among other things, it reflects how supported you feel for being who you are and how you have learned to face challenges. The mind-body connection becomes obvious when, on occasion, I am helping people improve their walking pattern and they become tearful, agitated, angry, disoriented, or exhausted. Even though this happens infrequently, it shows how habits of holding the body in a particular way can be deeply rooted in the psyche, often related to subconscious emotions and adaptive behavior patterns developed in childhood.

Improving the way you walk will ultimately be a relief, but it may feel foreign at first. Just as with standing, your brain may seem to prefer your familiar, habitual way of walking. You will need to make a point of changing the way you walk. This means consciously overriding your existing habits by intentionally following a new pattern of walking.

Understanding the ideas about how to walk will help, but the learning involved here is not intellectual; it is sensory-motor learning. In other words, you need time to sense and learn new ways of coordinating your movements, even if your mind understands what you are trying to do. Practicing the techniques in this book will gradually familiarize you with the new aspects of walking.

Now let's look at two areas of movement that will turn your good standing alignment into good walking practices: the feet and legs, and the pelvis and hips. An important point to remember: the following descriptions of what happens when you walk are referring to *walking barefoot*. Shoes have different heel heights and amounts of cushioning, which can alter the way you walk. Being barefoot is neutral and therefore the best way to practice any exercises for repatterning your gait.

THE FEET AND LEGS: WHAT HAPPENS WHEN YOU WALK

Many different actions happen in your legs and feet when you walk. To simplify this, consider there are two basic movements, occurring simultaneously: one leg is moving backward and the other leg is moving forward. Addressing these as two distinct movements makes it easier to learn the detailed actions of the legs and feet.

The Rear Leg and Foot

When you walk, the knee of one leg gradually straightens as that leg goes behind you. Straightening the knee causes the heel of the rear foot to press into the ground as your other leg goes forward. Explorations 16 and 17 will give you a sense of this. The rear heel needs to remain on the ground nearly until the front foot touches down. Keeping the rear heel down longer will improve your balance, which is a big advantage in improving your feeling of security. It may shorten the stride of your forward leg, but that is not a problem. It also may require changes in how you use your hip muscles and carry your pelvis, torso, and head. These will be discussed in greater detail later.

When the front foot is fully on the ground, the rear foot begins to leave the ground. The heel rises first, causing the foot to bend like a hinge at the ball of the foot, the padded part of the sole between the arch and the toes. This is where each toe connects to a *metatarsal* bone of the foot. When you walk, this area bends and straightens with each step, as shown in figure 3.1. You will have an opportunity to identify this hinge-like movement in Exploration 14. The ball of the rear foot is meant to bend fully just before the foot lifts off the ground and the rear leg is brought forward. This does not mean you should bounce off your toes when you walk. It means the sole of your foot needs to relax enough so that your weight follows through the entire length of your foot before it lifts off the ground. This means you will fully use your toes for balance.

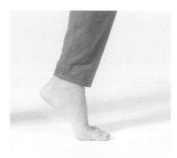

FIG. 3.1

The Forward Leg and Foot

With the ball of the foot bent like a hinge and the heel high off the ground, the rear foot is ready to lift up and move forward. The ankle of the rear leg needs to be relaxed when that foot comes off the ground. To get a sense of this, imagine your foot is dangling from your lower leg when you pick it up. This might cause you to bend your knee more than usual so that your foot doesn't drag on the floor when you bring it forward. Walking this way encourages the iliacus and psoas muscles to engage more fully.

While walking, the forward-moving foot lands in the vicinity of the midfoot, which includes the cuboid and the front of the calcaneus (see figure 2.11). This is near the balance point of the foot, which is roughly where you placed the dowel under your feet in Exploration 7. From there, your body weight balances along either side of the weight-bearing line, moving toward the space between the first and second toe. You will become more familiar with the weight-bearing line in Exploration 13.

Generally, the faster you walk or run, the farther forward you will land on your feet. If your feet touch down on the backs of your heels, it usually means that your body weight is too far behind your central vertical axis. People who walk with very heavy footsteps typically walk this way.

If your feet touch down approximately at the midfoot, you will feel that your feet are beneath you when you walk. You will also feel that the job of your legs is to *push* you forward. By contrast, if your feet touch down on the back of the heel, you will feel that your feet are far in front of you when you walk and that the job of your legs is to *pull* you forward. When it comes to walking, pushing is more efficient than pulling. You experience the feeling of pushing when you climb a steep hill and your legs must push into the ground to move you upward. When your alignment is balanced, the same feeling happens when walking on level ground, only to a lesser degree.

Another big advantage of your forward foot landing near the balance point is that it encourages your pelvis to maintain the proper tilt.

Exploration 13

- Sit on the front half of a chair with your knees bent and your feet flat on the floor. Imagine where the weight-bearing line is on the bottoms of both feet, extending diagonally from the outside half of your heel to the space between your first and second toes. Imagine that this line is drawn on the sole of each foot. See figure 2.11 (page 53).

- Slowly pick up both heels so that the balls of your feet bend, but your toes remain on the ground. As you do this, imagine that you are peeling the weight-bearing lines away from the floor, starting at your heels and moving toward the balls of your feet.

- Slowly reverse the movement, so your heels gradually return to the ground. As you do this, imagine that you are pressing the weight-bearing lines back into the floor.

- Repeat the same slow up-and-down movement for a few minutes. Remember, you are imagining a diagonal line, but your foot remains level. Do not tilt your foot inward when you lift your heel. The whole ball of your foot (inside and outside edges) should stay in contact with the floor.

- Stand up and walk for a minute. Can you imagine the same diagonal line on your feet as you walk? Feel if this alters the way you use your legs and hips when you walk.

The Pelvis and Hips: What Happens When You Walk

When you walk, your hips and pelvis naturally move a little bit in every direction over the course of each step. Let's briefly look at how the pelvis moves in each plane.

Side to Side
Walking mostly involves standing on one leg at a time, which also means lifting one leg at a time. The easiest way to do that is to take your weight off the leg before you lift it, and the easiest way to do that is to shift your weight onto the other leg. The easiest way to shift your weight is to relax the muscles in the buttock of the standing leg, so your pelvis shifts to that side. This is what you will feel in Exploration 14. I am not suggesting that you "swing your hips"; simply let your buttock muscles relax enough for your pelvis to move laterally in response to the weight shift from one leg to the other. If you do, it will feel like your leg bones, rather than your muscles, are holding you up.

You will notice that when your pelvis shifts to the side, your body weight is farther over the outside of your foot than the inside. This puts less pressure on the inside of the arch and more on the outside bones of the foot, which is where it belongs. If your feet hurt when you walk, make sure you pay attention to the side-to-side movement of your pelvis.

⩵ Exploration 14

- Stand with your feet parallel. Bend your left knee and raise your left heel, while keeping the ball of your foot on the ground. Relax your left foot so it bends easily at the ball. Lower your left heel back to the floor, then do the same thing with your right foot. Alternate between left and right until you can clearly feel the hinge motion at the ball of each foot. Relax the foot when you do this exercise, so the heel lifts because the knee lifts, not because you are pressing the ball of the foot into the ground.

- Shift your pelvis to the right so that your weight shifts onto your right leg. As you do, bend your left knee and keep your right knee straight. Next, shift your pelvis to the left so that your weight shifts onto your left leg; bend your right knee and keep your left knee straight. As you continue to shift slowly left and right, pay attention to the transfer of weight from one leg to the other. Feel how the lateral movement of your pelvis depends on relaxing the buttock muscles on the side toward which you are shifting. When this happens, notice how the outside of your foot carries more of your weight than the inside does.

- Now combine the two movements. When you shift your pelvis to the right, pick up your left heel. When you shift your pelvis to the left, pick up your right heel. Continue for another minute. This movement exaggerates the natural hip motion of walking.

Horizontal Trunk Rotation

As you walk, the knee of one leg straightens as that leg moves behind you. The gluteus and hamstring muscles need to engage for that knee to straighten. Exploration 15 isolates those muscles so you can clearly identify them through kinesthetic awareness. When those muscles work in conjunction with your back muscles, the result is a small but important rotation of your trunk (the combination of the pelvis, abdomen, back, and chest) toward the forward leg. You will feel this rotation in Explorations 16 and 17.

Trunk rotation is missing from the gait of most people I observe. This is a natural movement that twists the spine all the way up to the neck, performing an inner massage of the spinal muscles with every step. Trunk rotation results in the familiar walking pattern in which the opposite arm and leg move forward at the same time.

Excessive tension in the hip and lumbar muscles interferes with trunk rotation. Exercises 19 through 22 will help you sense what muscles control trunk rotation and what muscles need to relax to allow that rotation.

Pelvic Tilt

The tilt of pelvis needs to remain neutral while you walk, just as it does while you stand. As discussed in Chapter 2, a neutral tilt while standing occurs when the pelvis sits on top of the femoral heads. The majority of people will feel that this tilts their pelvis farther forward than usual. Carrying your pelvis this way does not mean holding it frozen in the "right" position, because it needs to be free to move when you walk. It is possible to maintain a neutral tilt even as your pelvis shifts from side to side and your trunk rotates laterally. You can experiment with tilting your pelvis forward and backward as you walk to feel how it affects the rest of your body, including your lumbar curve, the carriage of your head, the length of your stride, your legs and feet, and so on. Once you learn to sense your neutral pelvic tilt while sitting and standing, begin to practice it while you walk.

If your pelvic tilt is correct when you walk, you will feel a subtle springiness in your hip joints, as though you could easily bend your hip joints at any moment. This means your hips are not locked in the upright position. As you walk this way, you can imagine that your center of gravity has been lowered from your waist to your hip joints, as if those joints have gotten heavier. This sensation will help your body relax and improve your balance.

⚖ Exploration 15

- Lie facedown on the floor, and bend your right knee to a ninety-degree angle.

- Slowly raise your right thigh about five inches off the ground. Use your hand to feel how your buttock and thigh muscles have engaged to raise your leg. Relax your lower leg and knee muscles as much as you can. Bring your leg down and repeat 8 times.

- Repeat the same movements 8 times with your left leg. Again, sense how your buttock and upper leg muscles engage to lift your leg. These are the walking muscles that propel you forward with every step by straightening the rear knee.

⚖ Exploration 16

- Stand alongside a wall so that the wall is to your left. Place your left foot in front and your right foot behind, as if you were taking a long stride. Your left foot should be close to the wall, and both feet should be flat on the ground. Reach your right arm across your chest, and press your right hand into the wall. Bend both of your knees a little.

- Press your right heel firmly into the ground by straightening your right knee fully. Use the force of straightening that knee and pressing your heel down to rotate your trunk to the left, toward your forward leg. Simultaneously, use this trunk rotation to press your right hand more firmly into the wall. Do not bend or straighten your right elbow; feel how the force of your hand comes from your entire torso and your rear leg rather than from your arm alone. In other words, feel how pressing your right heel into the ground enables you to press your hand into the wall with greater force than if you just used your arm muscles.

- Return to the starting position and repeat the movement until you can easily feel that your trunk rotates as a result of pressing your heel down. Turn around so the wall is on your right, reverse the position of your legs, and try the same movement with your left hand pressing into the wall. Many people initially feel their trunk rotate *backward* when they straighten their rear leg, which is the opposite of what we are aiming for here. The exercises in this chapter will help you if you are having difficulty with this.

- Now, with your arms relaxed at your sides, once again straighten your rear leg and press your heel into the ground. Can you feel the same trunk rotation that you felt before, even though you are no longer reaching your arm across your chest? Repeat this until the feeling of your trunk rotating is familiar, with your legs in both positions.

- If you wish, place a tennis ball (or a similar small ball) under the back of the arch of your rear foot during the last movement. You will press into the ball as you straighten your rear knee. Having something to press your foot into may give you a clearer sense of how the heel presses into the floor—a feeling that many people have forgotten.

⌁ Exploration 17

- Start in a standing position. Take a step backward with your right leg, landing first on the ball of your foot and then on your heel. Feel how the buttock and thigh muscles engage as you straighten your right leg and press your heel down. At the same time, let your trunk rotate to the left (toward your forward leg). Look straight ahead, so your head does not turn with your trunk.

- Step backward with your left leg in the same fashion, pressing your heel down and rotating your trunk to the right. Continue looking straight ahead. This may be difficult to coordinate at first, so go slowly.

- Continue walking backward in this way for several minutes, until you can clearly sense the twisting in your waist and neck. Twisting is a natural part of walking, whether you're going backward or forward.

KEY POINTS OF WALKING (FOR THE LEFT BRAIN)

Let's look at the entire sequence of walking in a way that you can practice. When you walk, many things happen at the same time. The following steps attempt to separate the process into a manageable sequence of events, so you can relearn the natural pattern of walking. The timing of the actions suggested here may not be exactly what you feel when you practice. It depends on how fast you walk, as well as a number of other factors. I have taught these steps to many people, and they have proven to be very reliable. If you have difficulty with a certain movement, particularly trunk rotation, then practice the explorations and/or exercises associated with them.

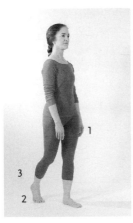

FIG. 3.2

Figure 3.2

1. Body weight shifts fully to the left leg: Exploration 14

2. The hinge at the ball of the right foot bends: Exploration 14; Exercise18

3. The right ankle is relaxed; Exploration 10

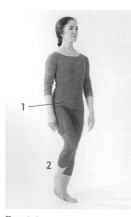

FIG. 3.3

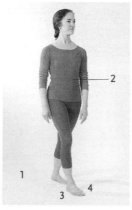

FIG. 3.4

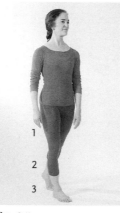

FIG. 3.5

Figure 3.3

1. The hip flexors engage to bend the right hip, bringing the right knee forward and up: Exercises 11 and 12

2. The right ankle is relaxed: Exploration 10

Figure 3.4

1. The left knee straightens out behind, pressing the left heel into the ground: Explorations 15–17; Exercises 19–22

2. The action of the left leg, hip, and back muscles causes the trunk to rotate to the right: Explorations 15–17; Exercises 19–22

3. The right foot touches down somewhere between the heel and midfoot: Exploration 7

4. Body weight travels through the right foot along the diagonal weight-bearing line: Exploration 13

Figure 3.5

1. Body weight shifts fully to the right leg: Exploration 14

2. The hinge at the ball of the left foot bends: Exploration 14; Exercise 18

3. The left ankle is relaxed: Exploration 10

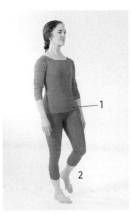

FIG. 3.6

Figure 3.6

1. The hip flexors engage to bend the left hip, bringing the left knee forward and up: Exercises 11 and 12

2. The left ankle is relaxed: Exploration 10

Figure 3.7

1. The right knee straightens out behind, pressing the right heel into the ground: Explorations 15–17; Exercises 19–22

2. The action of the right leg, hip, and back muscles causes the trunk to rotate to the left: Explorations 15–17; Exercises 19–22

3. The left foot touches down somewhere between the heel and midfoot: Exploration 7

4. Body weight travels through the left foot along the diagonal weight-bearing line: Exploration 13

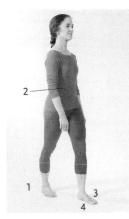

FIG. 3.7

EVEN SIMPLER KEY POINTS (FOR THE RIGHT BRAIN)

Maybe the preceding steps involve too many details for your liking. After all, you didn't originally learn to walk by following written instructions or thinking about it. Here is another option that may work better for you. You can practice the following list of suggestions while you walk. Each element is a piece of the whole walking pattern. Practice one at a time as you walk. Every few minutes switch to another element. If you find yourself unable to feel or imagine any of the suggestions, then skip them and work with the ones you can follow easily. Over time, most or all of them will feel natural.

1. Breathe.
2. Feel the ball of your rear foot bend like a hinge before you pick it up. Feel your toes pressing into the ground.
3. Relax your ankle when you pick up your foot. Imagine that your foot is dangling from your lower leg.
4. When your forward foot touches the ground, don't brace your hips and legs for impact. Instead, relax your hip muscles and imagine that your bones are doing all the work.
5. Relax your foot as it lands softly on the ground.
6. Imagine that each foot is traveling along its weight-bearing line.
7. Feel your rear knee straighten completely before picking up your heel, which presses your foot into the ground.
8. Keep your rear heel on the ground until your trunk rotates toward your forward leg.
9. Balance your head on top of your spine without holding it still. Let it move a little.

WALKING EXERCISES

These exercises take the alignment principles you learned in Chapter 2 and add the leg and trunk movements necessary for walking. The neutral pelvic tilt, the natural lumbar curve, and the upright head carriage all reinforce efficient actions of the leg and trunk muscles in walking. Remember, what applies to walking applies to running too.

18. TOE STRETCH

Prerequisite
Exploration 14

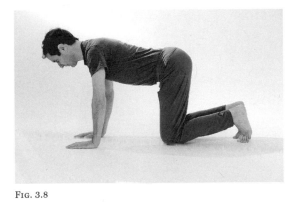

FIG. 3.8

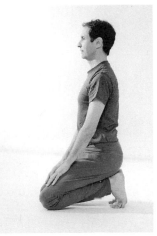

FIG. 3.9

Objective

To stretch the *plantar fascia* (the connective tissue in the arch of the foot) so you can bend the hinge at the ball of each foot more easily.

Position

▸ Kneel on all fours. Press the undersides of your toes and the balls of your feet into the ground (figure 3.8).

▸ Gradually shift your weight backward until your trunk is upright and your buttocks are resting on your heels (figure 3.9). If this is too painful, shift backward only as far as you can tolerate. Remain in this position for up to 1 minute.

Sensing

Feel the hinge of each foot bending as you relax the soles of your feet. Many people have not felt their feet bend this way for decades, so they need to approach this position slowly and gradually. Even if you can only tolerate it for 2 seconds, begin there and patiently increase the time as it becomes bearable. Flexibility in these joints will greatly improve your walking.

19. SUPINE HIP EXTENSION

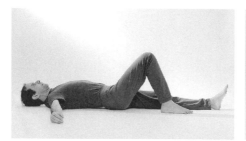

FIG. 3.10

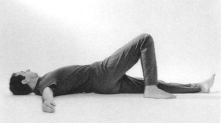

FIG. 3.11

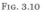

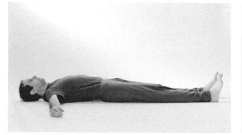

FIG. 3.12

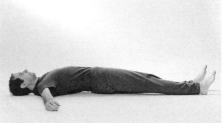

FIG. 3.13

Prerequisite
Exploration 15

Objective
To feel how engaging the thigh and buttock muscles on one side causes the pelvis to rotate toward the opposite side. This is directly applicable to trunk rotation in walking.

Part One: Position
- Lie on your back with your left leg straight and your right knee bent so the sole of your right foot is on the ground (figure 3.10).
- Press your right foot into the floor enough so that the right side of your pelvis lifts up; relax your back muscles. Feel how you are using the muscles in your right buttock to press your right foot down. When your pelvis lifts up on the right side, you will roll to the left; the left

side of your pelvis remains on the floor (figure 3.11). Relax and return to the starting position.

- ▶ Repeat this movement at least 8 times, then reverse legs and repeat the same action with your left leg.

Part Two: Position

- ▶ Lie flat on your back with your legs straight (figure 3.12).
- ▶ Pull your entire right leg down into the floor. Since the floor does not move, your leg will not go very far. However, if you relax your lower back, you will feel the right side of your pelvis lift a little. This is similar to the movement in Part One, but your pelvis will not move nearly as much because your knee is straight (figure 3.13).
- ▶ Relax and return to the starting position. Repeat the same action with your left leg, feeling how the left side of your pelvis lifts a bit. Alternate slowly between your right and left legs, relaxing for a second in between; repeat 8 times on each side.

Sensing

In both parts of this exercise, feel how the movement is caused by the muscles in your buttock and upper thigh rather than by the muscles near your knee or in your lower leg. Sense how your lumbar muscles need to relax sufficiently to allow your pelvis to move up on one side and roll toward the other. Feel how the buttock and leg muscles that press your foot or leg downward are not the same as the muscles that tense your lower back. This exercise mimics the actions of these muscles and the pelvis that occur when you walk.

20. Standing Trunk Rotation 1

Prerequisite
Explorations 14 and 16

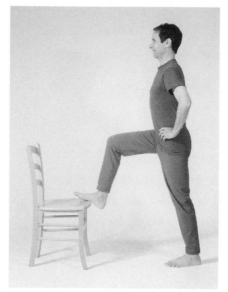

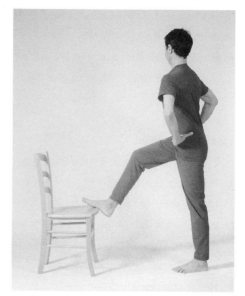

FIG. 3.14   FIG. 3.15

Objective

To relax the lower back muscles so the trunk can easily rotate right and left when it is moved by the legs.

Position

- ▶ Stand with your right foot on the edge of a chair and your right knee bent. Your left leg should be straight and slightly behind you. Rest your hands on your hips (figure 3.14). If balance is a problem, hold on to something with one hand for support.
- ▶ Slowly straighten your right knee, keeping your right foot in the same place. Keep your left leg stationary. The force of straightening your right leg will rotate your trunk backward on the right side (figure 3.15). You will need to relax your lower back muscles to allow this rotation. Relax your neck and keep your head facing forward.
- ▶ Return to the starting position by bending your right knee.
- ▶ Do the movement 8 times on your right side, then reverse legs and repeat 8 times on your left side.

Sensing

The goal here is to discover how to let your pelvis turn left and right with as little effort as possible. This will allow a lesser version of the same movement to happen naturally when you walk. If your pelvis is not moving, it means you are holding it in a fixed position. In this case, you need to feel *where* and *how* you are doing that, and learn how to release unnecessary tension in your back muscles.

21. Standing Trunk Rotation 2

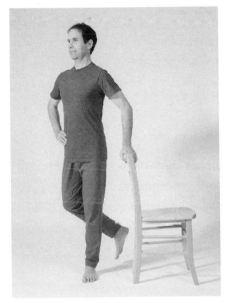 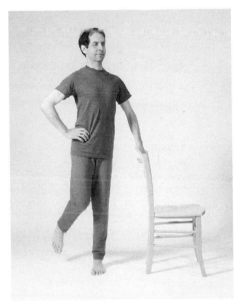

FIG. 3.16   FIG. 3.17

Prerequisite

Exploration 15

Objective

To improve the tone of the hip muscles involved in walking.

Position

▸ Stand on your left leg, with your right knee bent enough to bring your right foot off the floor. Place one hand on a chair or wall to help you keep your balance (figure 3.16). Rotate your trunk diagonally to the right.

▸ Using your left foot, leg, and hip muscles, rotate your trunk to the left, pivoting on your left leg. Keep your left knee straight, but don't hyperextend it. Rotate your trunk until it is facing diagonally to the left. Your left knee and foot remain facing straight ahead throughout the exercise (figure 3.17).

▸ Return slowly to the starting position. Perform this motion 8 times. Reverse legs and perform the same movements 8 times while standing on your right leg.

▸ When it is easy for you to do 8 repetitions, do the same movement without holding on to anything for balance. If you find this exercise particularly helpful, you may add another 1 to 2 sets (8 repetitions per set) to each side.

Sensing

Feel the buttock muscles of your standing leg work to move the opposite side of your pelvis forward. Sense how this action presses the foot of your standing leg into the floor. Encourage your foot to grasp the ground as your leg muscles work. Eventually, you will be able to do this movement without holding on to anything for support.

22. Standing Trunk Rotation 3

Prerequisites

Explorations 15–17

Objective

To feel how engaging the thigh and buttock muscles on one side causes the trunk to rotate toward the opposite side.

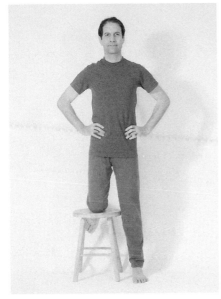

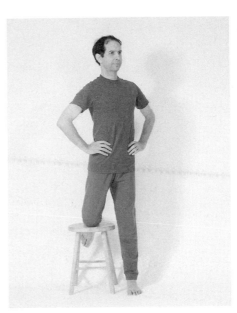

Fig. 3.18   Fig. 3.19

Position

▸ Place a stool close to a wall. Stand next to the stool on your left leg
  with your back to the wall. Bend your right knee and place your lower
  leg on the stool so that the sole of your right foot is against the wall
  (figure 3.18).

▸ Keeping your left leg stationary, press your right foot into the wall by
  using the muscles in your right buttock and leg (figure 3.19). Feel your
  trunk rotate to the left. Keep pressing your foot into the wall for a few
  seconds, then return to the starting position.

▸ Perform this movement 8 times, then reverse legs and repeat 8 times
  while standing on your right leg.

Sensing

Feel the muscles in your buttock and the back of your thigh engaging to
press your foot into the wall, which causes your trunk to rotate. These
are the walking muscles that propel you forward with each step. Feel how
the trunk rotation occurs without your back muscles making any effort.

Afterword

Y OU ARE NOW on your way to improving how you sit, stand, and walk. Remember, the primary purpose of these exercises is to remove the postural habits and dysfunctional movement patterns that interfere with your innate ability to carry yourself comfortably. In practical terms, this involves learning to relax muscles that are too tense, wake up muscles that have been inactive, and sense what good alignment feels like.

There is no absolute best order for addressing the many facets of improving your alignment. For example, some people have the best results if they first learn how to release their neck and carry their head, while others get the best results by learning how to release their lower back and carry their pelvis. The majority of people I have taught find it easiest and quickest to address sitting first, then standing, and then walking. This explains the order of the chapters in this book. If you have difficulty with an exercise, then look back in the book to find an earlier exercise or exploration of which you may not have gotten the full advantage or that you may have skipped completely.

When I work with people individually, one of my goals is often for them to be able to walk naturally and without pain. Usually we carry our standing postural habits with us when we walk, so I will address standing alignment before going into walking. Walking is important for all kinds of physiological and psychological reasons. Very few of my clients already use their legs and trunk to walk (or run) as I have suggested in this book. For these suggestions to feel right, your back muscles need to stop trying to hold you still while you walk, so walking the way I suggest has the additional benefit of teaching you how to relax your back. Walking then becomes a practical way to get exercise, calm your mind, and release tension from your muscles. For most people, it is very accessible; just go out the door and start walking.

Many people tell me they have trouble sitting all day long, yet that is what their job requires. I think our bodies get bored from sitting at a desk for hours on end, because there is very little movement to stimulate the nervous system. If our minds are occupied and our bodies are bored, then it is easy for our alignment to collapse, which is what Chapter 1 primarily addresses. This happens when we narrow our attention to the task at hand—for example, writing a book—and become unaware of our bodies and the space around us. This kind of prolonged focus is unnatural, even though many people experience it as normal. If you are sitting at a computer for long periods, take a break every hour or two; get up and walk around, look out a window as far into the distance as possible. If you consciously widen your field of vision for a few minutes, your eyes will relax.

When you return to your desk, begin by sitting the way you've learned from this book. Do a few of the sitting exercises if you need a reminder of how to get your pelvis back in the neutral position on the chair. Then remember to relax your eyes as you are looking at your computer. I have found the work of Les Fehmi to be helpful to many people in relieving the habit of focusing either their visual or mental attention too narrowly. His book, *The Open Focus Brain*, gives an excellent explanation of the pitfalls of this practice and offers effective mental exercises for regaining a more relaxed and open attention.

I have mentioned many times in this book that the body, mind, and psyche are not separate, challenging many people's unexamined assumption that they are unconnected fragments. Now I would like to go further and say that the body, mind, and psyche are the same thing viewed from different perspectives. The "thing" they are is you. Let me illustrate what

I mean. Imagine an apple on a table being experienced by four imaginary people who describe their perceptions. One person says he sees an apple. Another person says she sees a round red object. The third says he sees particles swirling around in a small spherical space. The last person says she smells a particular fragrance and tastes a particular sweetness. All of these people are describing the same thing from a different frame of reference.

Similarly, the words *body*, *mind*, and *psyche* are three ways of describing what you are. These words define different dimensions within you that are constantly interacting. The body, mind, and psyche interpenetrate each other in the same space. This is a more realistic way of seeing yourself than the conventional fragmented point of view. In particular, as you are trying to help your body feel better, consider that it constantly overlaps with your mind and psyche—which is why you need to pay attention to sensations and feelings.

The exercises in this book have helped many people eliminate pain. One reason is simply that the physics is reliable. Beyond this, however, is that the movements encourage a holistic way of addressing body alignment. In other words, they encourage you to experience your body, mind, and psyche as interconnected. I have observed that people who accept this approach typically recover more quickly and completely from pain problems than people who do not. This is not mere coincidence. Having an open view of yourself as a continuous interaction of sensations, thoughts, and feelings benefits the cells of the body. This is the inner environment in which relaxation, healing, and vitality can best exist.

Appendix

THE EXPLORATIONS in this book are designed to help you regain the kinesthetic awareness you need to do the exercises easily. The exact position of your body is not of primary importance in the explorations, and you will be able to do them easily by reading the written descriptions. However, it may be helpful for you to see the positions as well. They are all included in this appendix.

EXPLORATIONS 1, 2, AND 3

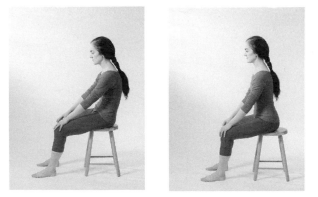

EXPLORATIONS 1–3

Exploration 4

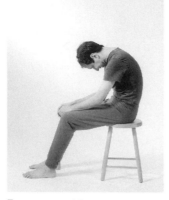

Exploration 4.1

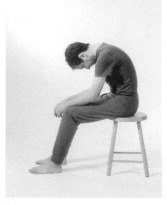

Exploration 4.2

Exploration 5

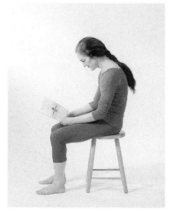

Exploration 5.1

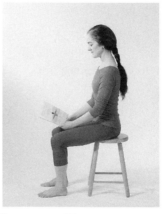

Exploration 5.2

EXPLORATION 6

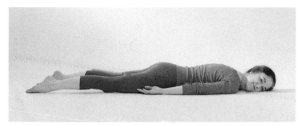

EXPLORATION 6.1

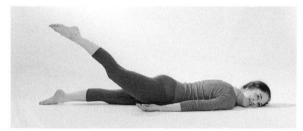

EXPLORATION 6.2

EXPLORATION 7

EXPLORATION 8

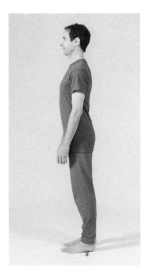

EXPLORATION 7

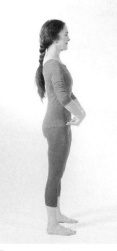

EXPLORATION 8.1

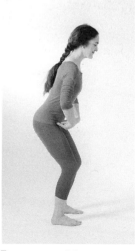

EXPLORATION 8.2

EXPLORATION 9

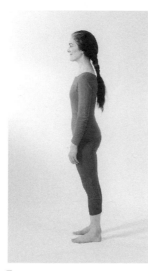

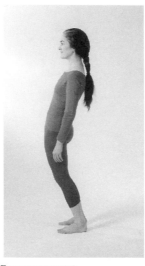

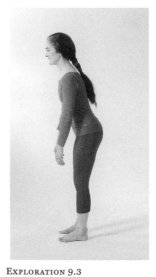

EXPLORATION 9.1

EXPLORATION 9.2

EXPLORATION 9.3

EXPLORATION 10

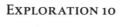
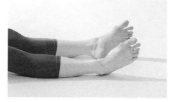

EXPLORATION 10.1

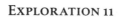
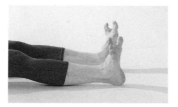

EXPLORATION 10.2

EXPLORATION 11

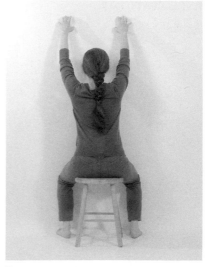

EXPLORATION 11

EXPLORATION 12

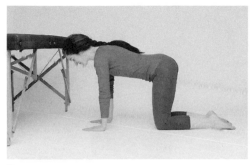

EXPLORATION 12.1

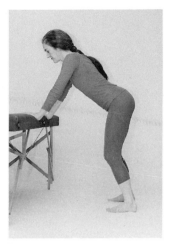

EXPLORATION 12.2

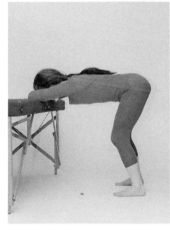

EXPLORATION 12.3

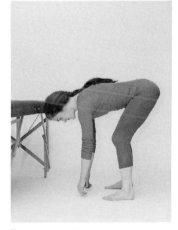

EXPLORATION 12.4

Exploration 13

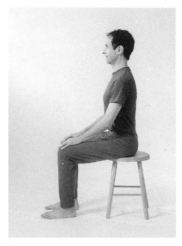

Exploration 13.1

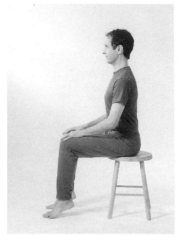

Exploration 13.2

Exploration 14

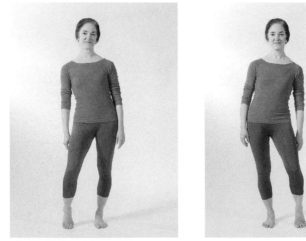

Exploration 14.1

Exploration 14.2

EXPLORATION 15

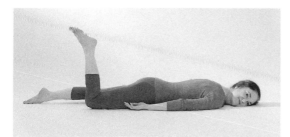

EXPLORATION 15.1

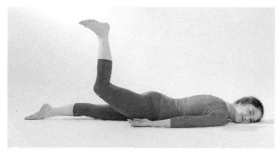

EXPLORATION 15.2

EXPLORATION 16

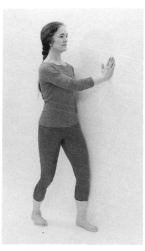

EXPLORATION 16.1

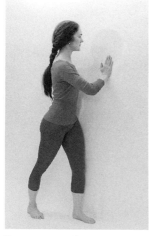

EXPLORATION 16.2

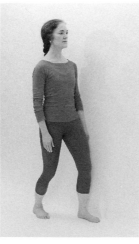

EXPLORATION 16.3

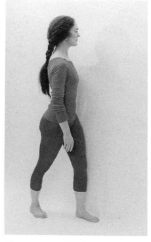

EXPLORATION 16.4

Exploration 17

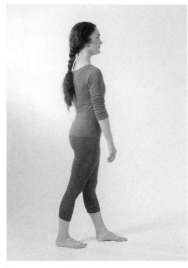

Exploration 17.1

Exploration 17.2

Also by Craig Williamson
Muscular Retraining for Pain-Free Living

I N THIS INNOVATIVE approach to eliminating chronic muscle pain, popular occupational therapist Craig Williamson reveals the roots of persistent pain and the simple, fundamental ways in which you can retrain your body for a pain-free life. *Muscular Retraining for Pain-Free Living* explains the basic principles behind Williamson Muscular Retraining, a pain-relief discipline, and offers a therapeutic exercise program that is practical and easy to understand. Common problems of poor posture, muscle tension, and stress-caused pain are corrected by seeing them through the lens of kinesthetic awareness (lacking in much of the population and typically overlooked by health-care practitioners). For anyone who wants to live a more healthy and comfortable life, *Muscular Retraining for Pain-Free Living* is an indispensable guide.